Dennis B. Worthen, PhD
Editor

The Millis Study Commission on Pharmacy
A Road Map to a Profession's Future

Pre-publication
REVIEWS,
COMMENTARIES,
EVALUATIONS . . .

"This work is important for all those interested in the history of pharmacy education. The editor and contributors have done a superb job of chronicling the key events subsequent to the Millis Commission report. There are still important issues to be resolved in terms of the evolution of the profession of pharmacy; this book clearly delineates the issues and outlines some of the steps that should take place to intertwine the missions of education, practice, and regulatory affairs."

James W. Cooper Jr., PhD, RPh, BCPS, CGP, FASCP, FASHP
Emeritus Professor and Consultant Pharmacist,
University of Georgia College of Pharmacy

"The Millis Study Commission's report was a much-anticipated and much-discussed landmark in pharmacy's continuing saga to transform itself. This book serves several purposes: It provides a historical perspective on the profession, an insider's view of the creation of the Millis report, and an analysis of the pharmacy profession's response to the report. It also provides valuable commentary on the still-unfinished task of aligning the professional aspirations of pharmacy with societal needs. The book will serve as a valuable resource for those engaged in current-day efforts to move the profession forward."

Randy P. Juhl, PhD
Vice Chancellor
and former Dean of Pharmacy,
University of Pittsburgh

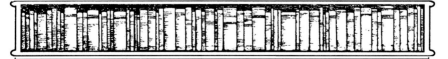

More pre-publication
REVIEWS, COMMENTARIES, EVALUATIONS . . .

"In the mid-1970s, pharmacy stood at a tipping point. Clinical pharmacy, a controversial approach to practice advocated by professional leaders for a decade, had gained sufficient acceptance among practitioners that a new general model for the future pharmacist was needed. The Millis Commission report, *Pharmacists for the Future*, took up the challenge and made the bold assertion that pharmacy was a knowledge system, not a distribution network. This book places the Study Commission's report in historical context and helps to explain how pharmacy evolved into its present position in American health care. The 1975 report still has much to say about pharmacy, and its reproduction in full in this book is a great service."

Gregory J. Higby, PhD, RPh
Executive Director,
American Institute of the History
of Pharmacy

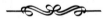

"The Millis Study Commission on Pharmacy laid the foundation for dramatic changes in pharmacy education and practice. Its report marked and solidified the shift of perspective and focus in pharmacy from the product to the patient. The Commission's approach to the profession from a pub-

lic interest perspective was unique and set the standard for subsequent examinations of the role of pharmacy in society. Although the final impact of the Commission is yet to be determined, this is an important historical analysis of its deliberations. Any student of current, evolving, pharmacy history will find this work of great interest. It details the inner workings and brings to life the behind-the-scenes activities of the Commission. The ideas put forth by the Commission related to pharmacy education and clinical practice have stood the test of time and are being implemented almost without exception.

This book is more than just a discussion of the work of the Commission; it also outlines the series of landmark events leading up to and following from the release of its report. The chapters in this book represent an accounting of events from a variety of perspectives. I was particularly fascinated by insights about Dr. John Millis. His personal views and comments by those who knew him well add a real depth to the publication. This book is a must-read for any educator or practitioner who wants to understand where the profession of pharmacy has come from and where it is going."

Holly L. Mason, PhD
Associate Dean for Academic Programs,
Purdue University School of Pharmacy
and Pharmaceutical Sciences

Pharmaceutical Products Press®
An Imprint of The Haworth Press, Inc.
New York • London • Oxford

The Millis Study Commission on Pharmacy

A Road Map to a Profession's Future

Pharmaceutical Products Press®
Titles of Related Interest

The Millis Study
Commission on Pharmacy
A Road Map
to a Profession's Future

Dennis B. Worthen, PhD
Editor

Pharmaceutical Products Press®
An Imprint of The Haworth Press, Inc.
New York • London • Oxford

For more information on this book or to order, visit
http://www.haworthpress.com/store/product.asp?sku=5151

or call 1-800-HAWORTH (800-429-6784) in the United States and Canada
or (607) 722-5857 outside the United States and Canada

or contact orders@HaworthPress.com

Published by

Pharmaceutical Products Press®, an imprint of The Haworth Press, Inc., 10 Alice Street, Binghamton, NY 13904-1580.

PUBLISHER'S NOTE
The development, preparation, and publication of this work has been undertaken with great care. However, the Publisher, employees, editors, and agents of The Haworth Press are not responsible for any errors contained herein or for consequences that may ensue from use of materials or information contained in this work. The Haworth Press is committed to the dissemination of ideas and information according to the highest standards of intellectual freedom and the free exchange of ideas. Statements made and opinions expressed in this publication do not necessarily reflect the views of the Publisher, Directors, management, or staff of The Haworth Press, Inc., or an endorsement by them.

Reprint edition of *A Road Map to a Profession's Future: The Millis Study Commission on Pharmacy* (Gordon and Breach Science Publishers, 1999).

.Cover design by Kerry E. Mack.

Library of Congress Cataloging-in-Publication Data

The Millis Study Commission on Pharmacy : a road map to a profession's future / Dennis B. Worthen, editor.
    p. cm.
    Originally published: A road map to a profession's future. Gordon and Breach, 1999.
    Includes bibliographical references and index.
    ISBN-13: 978-0-7890-2424-4 (hc. : alk. paper)
    ISBN-10: 0-7890-2424-1 (hc. : alk. paper)
    ISBN-13: 978-0-7890-2425-1 (pbk. : alk. paper)
    ISBN-10: 0-7890-2425-X (pbk. : alk. paper)
    1. Millis Study Commission on Pharmacy. 2. Pharmacy—Study and teaching. 3. Pharmacy—Vocational guidance. I. Worthen, Dennis B. II. Road map to a profession's future.
    [DNLM: 1. Study Commission on Pharmacy. Pharmacists for the future. 2. Education, Pharmacy—trends—United States. 3. History, 20th Century—United States. 4. Pharmaceutical Services—trends—United States. QV 18 R628 1999a]

RS122.5.R63 2005
615'.1'0973—dc22

2005015971 .

To Patti Lynn, my best friend and partner,
who first encouraged and supported the time
that we spent in Cleveland at Case Western Reserve University
and then encouraged and supported the development
of this undertaking

CONTENTS

ABOUT THE EDITOR

Dennis B. Worthen, PhD, is currently the Lloyd Scholar at the Lloyd Library and Museum in Cincinnati, OH. He is also an adjunct professor at the University of Cincinnati College of Pharmacy, where he teaches the history of pharmacy course. He retired from Procter & Gamble Health Care in 1999 after twenty-three years of service.

Dr. Worthen is the author of *Pharmacy in World War II* and the co-author (with Michael Flannery) of *Pharmaceutical Education in the Queen City: 150 Years of Service, 1850-2000,* a history of the University of Cincinnati College of Pharmacy. He is also the editor in chief of the *Dictionary of Pharmacy.* Dr. Worthen is a contributing editor for the *Journal of the American Pharmacists Association,* where he authors the series "Heroes of Pharmacy." He is also a contributing author for the *International Journal of Pharmaceutical Compounding.* In 1998, he was the founding co-editor of The Haworth Press's Pharmaceutical Heritage book series.

CONTRIBUTORS

Marie A. Abate is Professor of Clinical Pharmacy, Director of the West Virginia Center for Drug and Health Information, and Director of Assessment at West Virginia University School of Pharmacy. She received her BS in pharmacy and PharmD degrees from the University of Michigan.

Michael C. Shannon was Professor in the Division of Pharmacy Practice and Science, Director of Continuing Education, and Assistant Dean for Professional Affairs at the University of Kentucky. He received his BS in pharmacy at the University of Rhode Island, MS in the history of pharmacy at the University of Wisconsin, and PhD in continuing education also at the University of Wisconsin.

Lawrence C. Weaver is Professor and Dean Emeritus, College of Pharmacy, University of Minnesota. He received a BS in pharmacy from Drake University and a PhD in pharmacology at the University of Utah. He worked as a scientist in the pharmaceutical industry before returning to the University of Minnesota. He also served as Vice President of Pharmacy at the Pharmaceutical Manufacturers Association.

Albert I. Wertheimer is Director of the Center for Pharmaceutical Health Services Research, and Professor at Temple University School of Pharmacy, in Philadelphia. Previously, he has served as Director, Outcomes Research and Management, Merck & Company, Inc., Vice President at First Health, Dean and Associate Vice President of the Philadelphia College of Pharmacy and Science, and Department Chair and Director of Graduate Studies at the University of Minnesota. He earned a BS in pharmacy at the University of Buffalo and PhD from Purdue University, and was a postdoctoral fellow at St. Thomas' Hospital Medical School, University of London (UK).

Allen I. White was Professor and Dean Emeritus of the College of Pharmacy at Washington State University. He received his BS in pharmacy and his MS and PhD in pharmaceutical chemistry, all from the University of Minnesota.

Foreword to the New Edition

For me, the Millis Study Commission on Pharmacy has very personal significance. Not only do I now lead the organization that charged the Commission and published its work, but I also studied as a graduate student in the Kellogg Foundation–supported pharmaceutical clinical scientist program at the University of Minnesota. There I had the distinct privilege of coming to know Dr. Millis.

"Divine discontent"—this phrase must have been one of Jack Millis's most favored expressions. He used it as he was considering whether to accept the hands-on role as the working chair of the AACP Study Commission on Pharmacy in 1973. He continued to use the phrase as he chaired the National Advisory Committee of the Kellogg Program from 1979 through 1984. Were "we"—a profession in the first case and a group of graduate students in the latter—sufficiently dissatisfied with the status quo of pharmacists' service to society and the knowledge system it represented to embark on a period of profound change?

The decades since the original report was published have been remarkable in terms of the changes in pharmacy education and the differentiated roles that pharmacists assume today. This is a credit to the profession's many leaders who have a shared vision for pharmacy practice that is first and foremost patient centered. But what has changed most since the initial publication of the Millis Study Commission report is that medication use has assumed a much more central role in health care at all levels. Recognition is growing outside of pharmacy that medication-use specialists, those educated and licensed to practice pharmacy, are essential to the delivery of quality patient care.

With most of the observations and recommendations published in the report largely addressed, it would be easy to call for a new Millis Commission to embark on a study of medication use and pharmacy practice in the twenty-first century. What is most interesting is that the Institute of Medicine (IOM) is, in fact, about to embark on such an analysis taking the "outside looking in" approach of the Millis Commission even one step further.

I hope that "Pharmacists for the Future" and this book are among the resources the IOM study commission reviews as it sets about its work. These establish an important context for medication use and the role of pharmacists and shed light on the significant changes in both of these that occurred in the past century. Without such a valuable look back any attempt to look forward would be limited.

In that same vein, the original Study Commission Report and the interpretive materials contained in this book are important resources for pharmacy students, faculty, and practitioners as well. This book compiles so much of our history, strategic thinking, and forward progress as a profession—we are deficient if we fail to access it regularly to evaluate our future pathways.

Dennis Worthen and his co-authors deserve significant credit for keeping this important information in front of pharmacists and other stakeholders in medication use. Hopefully the "divine discontent" of contemporary leaders in health care will stimulate change that more effectively integrates the knowledge system of medication use and the important contributions of pharmacists into quality patient care that is safe and accessible for all.

Lucinda L. Maine, PhD
Executive Vice President
American Association of Colleges of Pharmacy

Foreword to the Original Edition

This book is an essential epilogue to the Millis Study Commission on Pharmacy. It is rare, indeed, that the work of such a commission can be reviewed in retrospect, regarding its real effects.

The importance of this volume is twofold: first, placement of the Millis Commission within the context of earlier studies that examined the responsibilities of pharmacy educators and the role of pharmacists; second, its reception by both educators and practitioners.

The Millis Commission was a significant landmark for pharmacy. It was a citizen's commission, not a pharmacy commission. Millis and his colleagues looked at pharmacy's evolving responsibilities to society and patients and its role as part of the health care system. Earlier studies had been internally focused—by pharmacists and for pharmacists. The Millis Study Commission marked a maturation of the profession and its willingness to become accountable to its users.

It may be another generation before the success or failure of the Millis Commission can be fully assessed. There have been both proponents and opponents to the recommendations in the final report, *Pharmacists for the Future.* However, it is interesting to note how many of the current efforts in pharmacy and pharmacy education reflect deliberations and recommendations of the Millis Commission. Perhaps the greatest contribution of the entire effort was the opportunity to articulate and focus a message for pharmacists of the future—it's the patient!

It is unlikely this book would have been published if not for the zeal of Dr. Dennis Worthen. The work is basic for anyone who would understand what has happened and is happening to those who practice the profession of pharmacy and those who teach those practitioners.

In his Preface, Worthen suggests there are three groups for whom this book is relevant (that is not what *he* says, but rather my interpretation):

1. Those who believe the Commission and its efforts were responsible for the current exciting events in clinical pharmacy practice and pharmaceutical care.
2. Those who believe the Commission could have done much more.
3. Those who have little idea about the Commission, the efforts of those who worked with it, and its ultimate effects on pharmacy.

This book has something for all three groups, but could be most beneficial to the third group.

I never met John Millis, but his work and dedication are beautifully served by Dennis Worthen and his collaborators.

Mickey C. Smith, PhD
F.A.P. Barnard Professor of Pharmacy Administration
Professor of Marketing and Management
School of Pharmacy, University of Mississippi

Preface

During the preparation of this work, I talked to a large number of pharmacy educators about the Millis Study Commission on Pharmacy and its impact on the profession. Responses and reactions were quite varied, as might be expected. Some were very positive and thought that the Commission was successful, but there was not just one area where success was noted. Many, especially younger educators, had never read the final report, *Pharmacists for the Future.* Although they had heard about the Millis Commission, their perspectives were, at best, secondhand. Finally, there were those who thought the Commission was a failure. Some because of the process used, some because of the lack of specific mandates emerging from the Commission's work, and some "just because."

As I listened to the various responses, especially the negative ones, I formed an analogy that I thought represented the reactions well. It goes as follows: Imagine leaving home early one day to drive to the mountains. After a full morning's drive, the mountains appear no closer—they still hang on the horizon. The journey continues throughout the afternoon, but still the mountains appear no closer. We wonder when, and if, we will ever arrive. Finally, we turn and look back, only to discover that we have moved so far that we can no longer see our starting point. While the goal has not yet been reached, the journey to get there was well begun.

The Commission met from September 1973 to September 1975 and its report, *Pharmacists for the Future,* was released in December 1975. The impact of the Commission is still being debated. There are those who see it as the engine, or driver, of change that the profession has been undergoing for the past twenty years. Others see the Commission as having fallen short of its charge and the profession's expectations. There is also a third group, those who have little idea or knowledge about the Commission; they should have an understanding, however. Pharmacy, and its practitioners, must be learning and changing constantly if it is to meet the needs of the society it is part of and is dedicated to serve.

Several of the contributors to this work knew Dr. Millis. Larry Weaver was part of the AACP leadership group that commissioned the study, as was Al White. Albert Wertheimer was one of the architects, along with Larry Weaver, who developed a graduate program designed to implement some of the recommendations of the Commission. My personal reason for the book was Jack Millis himself. I was a returning graduate student at Case Western Reserve University while the Commission was meeting. Working in the area of drug information, I had many opportunities to have contact with Dr. Millis. Only recently have I really understood the influence he had on me.

This work is not intended as an exhaustive examination or critical history of the Millis Study Commission on Pharmacy. Instead, it is a series of perspectives that are designed to place the Commission in the context of what came before and what happened after. It is still too early for a full history to be written, especially if it has as part of its charge to examine the impact the Commission had on the profession of pharmacy and the educational process for its practitioners. The relevance of the Commission to professional change can best be understood when one considers what preceded it, what triggered it, and how it chose to approach its charge.

Acknowledgments

I would like to acknowledge and thank the many individuals who have been helpful in the development and preparation of this work.

- The American Institute of the History of Pharmacy, especially its director, Greg Higby, and the staff of the Wisconsin State Archives were gracious and helpful in working with the records of the American Association of Colleges of Pharmacy.
- The staff of the Archives at Case Western Reserve University assisted in the use of the papers of John S. Millis.
- The American Association of Colleges of Pharmacy and its executive vice president, Richard P. Penna, granted permission to reproduce the final report, *Pharmacists for the Future*. Thanks also to The Haworth Press and Mickey C. Smith, who gave permission to reprint the Millis materials from the *Journal for Pharmacy Teaching,* as well as Lucinda Maine, who granted permission to reprint this compilation.
- And finally, I am indebted to all of the individuals, even those who questioned the ultimate success of the Study Commission, who graciously and patiently responded to my numerous questions.

Introduction

The Workings of the Commission

Dennis B. Worthen

In his presidential address to the American Association of Colleges of Pharmacy (AACP) in 1971, Arthur E. Schwarting presented his vision for a new study and evaluation of pharmacy and pharmaceutical education. Schwarting cited the lack of "insight and foresight" of the future role of pharmacists in the health care system as the basis for this proposal. The stated objectives of the study were to

1. identify the needs of society for appropriate drug therapy and related pharmaceutical services and acknowledge the deficiencies in health care as they relate to these services;
2. identify role models to fulfill these needs in concert with the functions of other health professionals;
3. define the nature and structure of future programs to educate these practitioners;
4. define the manner by which these findings should be implemented.[1]

Dean Schwarting formed an AACP committee of himself, Jere E. Goyan, John A. Biles, George P. Hagar, and William J. Kinnard Jr. to obtain funding, find a chairperson, and develop the final charge for the study.

The committee contacted a number of individuals to obtain insights on both the proposed study and the development of a short list for a potential chair. These discussions followed a predetermined outline. Some of the questions were to obtain

1. an expression of your feeling regarding the feasibility and significance of the proposed commission study;

2. your opinion regarding the usual processes for establishing a commission. Who should foster the study? (Public or private enterprise, American Council on Education, Institute of Medicine of the National Academy of Science, etc.); and,
3. how should the commission be represented? What should be the organizational structure? What individuals should be considered for (a) membership, (b) chairman of the commission?[2]

Jere Goyan prepared a paper, "A Case for a Study of Pharmacy Practice and Pharmacy Education," as the starting point for discussion with potential commission chairs. Schwarting's charge to the commission was based on the sum and substance of this document:

1. an evaluation of the system of pharmacy service in the whole structure of health care;
2. an evaluation of recent and current changes in pharmacy education and continuing education; and
3. a determination of the nature and extent of drug misuse in the present system of health care.[3]

John S. Millis, then president of the National Fund for Medical Education (NFME), was identified as the best and leading candidate for chair. In addition to his role at NFME, Millis had chaired successful commissions on the graduate education of physicians and one on dietetics. He had also served as the chair of President Nixon's Panel on Heart Disease. A physicist by education, he became president of Western Reserve University in 1949 where he remained until his retirement in 1967. His retirement coincided with a major accomplishment of his presidency, the federation of Western Reserve and Case Institute of Technology to form Case Western Reserve University.

Millis was forthright in his responses about how to form and operate the proposed commission. He believed that a commission made up of representatives of the vested interest groups of a convening body was a mistake. This approach was frequently marred by political compromise and the need to protect the status quo. He pointed out, even in these early discussions with the AACP committee, that a representative body could result in the lack of consensus and minority reports. Instead, he advocated the establishment of the commission as a citizens' group, with the public as its primary interest. He believed that this approach, which had been used in both the graduate medical education and the dietetics commissions, was a large part of their success.[4]

Millis, the man, was very much in evidence during his discussions with the AACP committee. He was direct to a fault. During the October 23, 1972, meeting he explained his working style.

> Chairman of the Commission will assume major staff responsibility. My style is to be the staff in a very real sense. I don't use ghost writers. I write my own stuff. I learn from talking to people face to face. Most commissions operate with a chairman presiding over the meeting and he hopefully assigns staff to write, I write my own reports and don't fuss around.[5]

In October 1972, AACP invited Millis to serve as chair and form a commission. The first items in the "Points of Understanding Re: A Commission on Pharmacy" addressed the nature of the commission itself.

1. to be formed at the request of the American Association of Colleges of Pharmacy;
2. to be an independent body;
3. to be viewed as "in the public interest," studying pharmacy as a profession whose members serve the "public interest" through the practice of a health vocation and profession;
4. to render its report to
   a. the AACP
   b. the pharmacy profession
   c. the universities
   d. the health professions
   e. the public.[6]

Millis wanted thinkers and learners on the Commission. He was up front with his intention to forego individuals who would be seen as representing a particular segment of pharmacy. Instead, he insisted that they

> be selected on the basis of their individual demonstrated commitment to the public welfare as it is affected by health service, for recognized capacity for learning and judgment, and for expertise in relevant areas of knowledge and professional activity.

The work of this body was conceived to be as a "group learning" experience and not as the political resolution of conflicting points of view and of vested interests. The work of the chairman is conceived as the identification and the foundation of specific matters, areas and problems to be studied, the identification of groups and individuals to be consulted by the commission; the preparation of working and of position papers; and the usual activities required of a chairman of a study group.[7]

The members of the Commission were:

John Biles, Dean, School of Pharmacy, University of Southern California

Robert Chalmers, Associate Dean and Professor, School of Pharmacy and Pharmacal Sciences, Purdue University

Leighton Cluff, Professor and Chair, Department of Medicine, College of Medicine, University of Florida

Henry F. DeBoest, Vice President, Corporate Affairs (retired), Eli Lilly (died before the third meeting of the Commission)

Bryce Douglas, Vice President, Research and Development, Smith Kline & French

Jan Koch-Weser, Associate Professor of Pharmacology, Harvard Medical School and Chief of Clinical Pharmacology Unit, Massachusetts General Hospital

John S. Millis, Chairman, National Fund Medical Education and Chancellor Emeritus, Case Western Reserve University

Victor Morgenroth Jr., Community Pharmacist

Charles E. Odegaard, Professor of Higher Education and President Emeritus, University of Washington

Rozella Schlotfeldt, Professor of Nursing, Frances Payne Bolton School of Nursing, Case Western Reserve University

William E. Smith Jr., Director, Pharmacy and Central Services, Memorial Hospital Medical Center

Robert Straus, Professor and Chairman, Department of Behavioral Science, College of Medicine, University of Kentucky

Once the Commission was formed and Millis appointed chair, the first order of business was to secure funding. Millis became active in helping AACP approach various foundations and making the case for the significance of the study. Because of his work on previous commissions and his years of academic leadership he was well-known and highly regarded. The first funding was provided by the American Foundation for Pharmaceutical Education (AFPE). This allowed Millis time to develop the starting point for the Study Commission and to gain additional insights on pharmacy and its place in the health care system. Additional funding support came from the W. K. Kellogg Foundation, The Commonwealth Fund, The Edna McConnell Clark Foundation, and the Robert Wood Johnson Foundation. With funding secure, Millis was ready to start the actual work of the Study Commission in the fall of 1973.

In August 1973, Millis provided his initial thoughts on the charges to the Commission. The general priorities established the themes that would resound during its working life.

> Since the Commission has been formed at the request of the American Association of Colleges of Pharmacy, its Report and Recommendations must deal directly with the education of pharmacists. The report must answer such questions as:
> Who should be educated?
> How many should be educated?
> How should they be educated?
> For what should they be educated?
> By far the most important question in this list is the last one—"For what should they be educated?"
>
> This leads to the thought that, though the resolution of questions about pharmacy education is the basic responsibility of the Commission, the starting point for the inquiry is the examination of such questions as:
> What do pharmacists do?
> What can pharmacists do?
> What should pharmacists do?
> In what settings, organizations, and/or institutions should pharmacists work?
> How is the work of the pharmacist related to the work of other health professionals?

How should the services of pharmacists be valued economically?[8]

The design of the Study Commission was for the group to sit as a committee of the whole. Discussion and learning was approached as a team. Discussion, debates, and insights were shared from the multiple areas of expertise and the various perspectives represented by the individual members.

The Study Commission invited a number of individuals and organizations to consult with it. These were grouped to provide both individual and organizational perspectives and agendas. Thus, there were meetings with pharmacy practitioners, regulators on both the national and state levels, pharmaceutical manufacturers, physicians, pharmacy educators, and others representing the health care system. Over the life of the Commission, eighty-one individuals appeared. (A complete list including addresses and affiliations appears at the end of the report, *Pharmacists for the Future.* Appendix A.)

The process for each Commission meeting was fairly standard. A stenotypist recorded every meeting; he would make two copies of the typed transcript, sending one to Millis in Cleveland and the other to the secretary, Lucy Joutz, at AACP headquarters. The Study Commission would hear the presentations by the consultants and there was time for considerable discussion, first with consultants and then among Commission members only. Millis would use the transcript and Mrs. Joutz's notes to prepare summaries, or précis, of the meetings; the précis and minutes would be provided to Commission members. At the next meeting, there would be a discussion to correct or clarify these summaries. The précis were used both as a reference and as the basis for preparation of the final report.

The Commission finished its work at the September 1975 Cleveland meeting, when the group voted to adjourn. While this date represented the end of the formal work of the Study Commission, it also marked the beginning of the recommendation for the education of future pharmacists as set out in the report, *Pharmacists for the Future,* presented to the public in Washington, DC, on December 5.

After completion of the Commission's work, Millis again articulated his vision and rationale for choosing members based on their ability to think and learn rather than for their affiliation with a particular view or organization. He stated his belief that when commissions made up of representatives of the interest groups succeeded, it was because of compromise, not wisdom. He felt that this approach produced the lowest common denominator of prejudice rather than the highest order of wisdom. He addressed the issue of consensus using the approach of a group of intelligent learners.

> We never had to call for a vote, never gather a minority report. Every conclusion was arrived at by going through the common learning experience from our separate points of view, background and experiences. I feel the report does represent the finest we could produce, with our human frailty, and represents the highest multiple of our individual wisdom.[9]

NOTES

1. A.E. Schwarting, "Address of the President: Some Propositions for Progress," *Am. J. Pharm. Educ., 36,* 351 (1972).

2. John Biles, "Letter to John S. Millis," August 24, 1972, University Archives, Case Western Reserve University, Classification # 1DD9, Box 41, Folder 6.

3. University Archives, Case Western Reserve University, Classification # 1DD9, Box 41, Folder 6.

4. American Association of Colleges of Pharmacy Papers in the American Institute of History of Pharmacy Collection at the State Historical Society of Wisconsin, Madison, WI, Mss # 293, Box 166, Folder 6.

5. American Association of Colleges of Pharmacy Papers in the American Institute of History of Pharmacy Collection at the State Historical Society of Wisconsin, Madison, WI, Mss # 293, Box 165, Folder 10.

6. A. Schwarting, "Attachment to Letter to J. Millis," October 16, 1972, University Archives, Case Western Reserve University, Classification # 1DD9, Box 41.

7. J.S. Millis, "Memorandum for Dean Schwarting Concerning the Proposed Study Commission on Pharmacy," November 22, 1972, University Archives, Case Western Reserve University, Classification # 1DD9, Box 41.

8. J.S. Millis, "Memorandum to Members of the Study Commission on Pharmacy," August 13, 1973, University Archives, Case Western Reserve University, Classification # 1DD9, Box 42.

9. J.S. Millis, "Kremers Lecture, University of Wisconsin School of Pharmacy," March 11, 1976, University Archives, Case Western Reserve University, Classification, Personal Papers, File A-89-008.

Chapter 1

Transitions: Changing Emphases in Pharmacy Education, 1946 to 1976

Michael C. Shannon

INTRODUCTION

In 1971, then president of the American Association of Colleges of Pharmacy (AACP), Arthur Schwarting, called for the creation of a Commission to "determine the scope of pharmacy services in health care and project the educational processes necessary to insure that these services are obtained."[1] The Study Commission on Pharmacy (Millis Commission) was formed in the fall of 1972 with John S. Millis, PhD, chancellor emeritus of Case Western Reserve University, as chairperson. The results of that study were reported in *Pharmacists for the Future: The Report of the Study Commission on Pharmacy* (Appendix A).[2]

The Millis Commission was the latest in a line of seventeen studies of pharmacy that had been conducted or proposed through 1976, and the third major study conducted between 1917 to 1976.[3] Moreover, the Millis Commission was quite different in character and focus than the previous two major studies, the Charters Study (1924-1927)[4] and *The Pharmaceutical Survey* (1946-1949).[5] The surveys and studies conducted up to the 1960s could be characterized as internally focused, often task analysis driven, and based on data coming from pharmacy and pharmacy-related sources. We might characterize the studies after 1960 as externally focused, using data both from within and from outside the profession, and more system oriented than their earlier counterparts (Table 1.1). By the time of the Millis Commission, for example, it was clear that the country had a major problem with drug abuse and misuse.[6] It was also clear to the mem-

TABLE 1.1. Conferences and Studies on Pharmacy Conducted Between 1949 and 1976

Year	Conference/Study
1961	Survey of Retail Pharmacists; conducted by Benson & Benson, Inc., Princeton, NJ, for the Reader's Digest, October 1961.
1963	Mirror to Hospital Pharmacy by the American Society of Hospital Pharmacists.
1965	Exploratory Paper for a Proposed National Study of Pharmacy As a Professional Occupation by Glenn A. Sonnedecker for the American Pharmaceutical Association.
1967	Pharmacy-Medicine-Nursing Conference on Health Education at the University of Michigan.
1967	The Task Force on Prescription Drugs.
1970	Proposed Study of Pharmaceutical Education's Immediate and Long-Range Responsibilities in Comprehensive Health Care.
1970	Invitational Conference on Pharmacy Manpower by the National Center for Health Services Research and Development and the University of California.
1972	Conference on Interrelationships of Educational Programs for Health Professionals sponsored by the Institute of Medicine.
1973	Communicating the Value of Comprehensive Pharmaceutical Services to the Consumer by the Dichter Institute for Motivational Research, Inc.
1973	Study of Costs of Educating Health Professionals by the Institute of Medicine, National Academy of Science.

Source: Adapted from W. Skinner, "Summary of Selected Surveys and Conferences Concerning Pharmacy." Unpublished manuscript (42 pp.). University Archives, Case Western Reserve University, Classification # 1DD9, Box 43, Folder 1.

bers of the Millis Commission that they were dealing with a health care delivery system that, in addition to pharmacists and pharmacy, included other health care professionals, institutions, and organizations.[7]

How did the changes in perspective represented in the Millis Commission and its report come to be? What changes had occurred in pharmacy education, pharmacy practice, and pharmacy as a profession? How great were the changes that had occurred in the "world at large" and what impact did those changes have on the work of the Millis Commission? We will try to answer those questions as this chapter unfolds. First, however, we need to establish our time frame. The Elliott Survey was inaugurated on April 15, 1946.[8] The recommendations were provided to AACP and other appropriate pharmacy organizations well in advance of the actual publication of its report, *The Pharmaceutical Survey,* in 1950.[9] The Millis Commission actually started meeting in 1973, and the report was published in late 1975 and not widely available until 1976. The changes occurring in the thirty years between the beginning of the Elliott Survey and the publication of the Millis Commission report will be examined.

THIRTY YEARS OF CHANGE

There were profound changes in the world during the thirty years between 1946 and 1976, in the United States, in health care, and in pharmacy. It is not the purpose of this chapter to chronicle the events of the world between 1946 and 1976; nevertheless, it would be useful to get a sense of the times and the sensibilities that permeated this period. Any attempt to select important events from the past and/or to interpret those events as they relate to specific topics is a recipe for controversy, particularly when one is considering events that are only thirty to sixty years old. Yet we want to give a snapshot of life in the United States during this thirty-year period. At the risk of leaving out one or more occurrences of importance to some, we will try to capture the flavor of the times (Table 1.2). However, many events in the world at large had tremendous impact on the delivery of health care and on the professionals providing that care. Major advances in medicine, health care, and pharmacy that occurred during those years will be covered in this section.

Reflecting the desire to provide an overview rather than write a detailed history of the period, our narrative will be simple and straightforward. The simplest perspective would see the period as two minieras that can be identified but not completely separated. The "good life–American dream" era was predominant in the early years, and it merged with an "alienation-rebellion" era that was dominant in the later years of the period. The threads making up the fabric of these minieras were not always easy to see, particularly the beginnings of them. Yet the fabrics existed and continue to exist in the American psyche. Let's see how we can capture the flavor of times.

TABLE 1.2. Thirty Years of Change

Year	Health Care Mileposts	Societal Mileposts
1946	Elliott Commission established	Emergence from WWII with "good life" and "American dream" motifs
1947	Tetracycline discovered	Male sexual behavior explored by Kinsey
		Baseball integrated as Jackie Robinson and Larry Doby join majors
1948	Chloramphenicol discovered	Creation of Israel
1949	Elliott Commission Report issued	"Fair Trade" legislation passed in forty-nine states
1951		Rock music era begins
1952	Durham-Humphrey Amendments to 1938 Food and Drug Act	Eisenhower elected president
1953	*Rauwolfia serpentina* marketed	CIA helps shah to power in Iran
		Female sexual behavior explored by Kinsey
1954	Chlorpromazine marketed	Civil rights legislation passes Congress
		Separate but equal approach to desegregation overthrown by Supreme Court
		Hydrogen bomb exploded
		Dien Bien Phu falls—United States gets more involved in Vietnam
1955	Polio vaccine (Salk) available	Rosa Parks rides in front of bus
1956		Counterculture era begins
		Peyton Place published
		Eisenhower reelected president
1957		Sputnik satellite launched by Russia
1959		Cuba falls to Fidel Castro
1960	Five-year curriculum begins in pharmacy schools except in California	Kennedy elected president
		TV brings politics into mainstream America
	Birth control drugs become available	U-2 spy plane shot down by Russia
1961	Ampicillin marketed	
1962	Effectiveness of drug product required by FDA amendments	Cuban missile crisis
	Methyldopa marketed	

TABLE 1.2 *(continued)*

Year	Health Care Mileposts	Societal Mileposts
1963	Drug abuse appears as national issue	Kennedy assassinated
	Atromid S marketed	
	Valium marketed	
1964	Propranolol marketed	Gulf of Tonkin Resolution gets U.S. deeply into Vietnam
		Johnson elected president—starts Great Society programs
1967	Medicaid/Medicare legislation passed	Medicaid/Medicare legislation passed
	Clinical pharmacy era begins	Vietnam protests reach peak
	CE for pharmacists becomes mandatory in Florida and Kansas	
	Third-party payment for Rxs begins in Michigan	
1968	Health care accountability era begins	Johnson declines to run for president
		Nixon elected president
		Kennedy (RFK) assassinated
		Martin Luther King assassinated
1969		Man lands on the moon
1970	Controlled Substances Act passed	
1972	ASHP leaves APhA umbrella	Watergate break-in
1973	DEA created	
1974	Michigan passes product selection legislation	Nixon resigns/Ford becomes president
1975	Millis Commission Reports	
1976	NABPLEX examination first given	Bicentennial of nation celebrated
		"Fair Trade" laws made irrelevant by national legislation

What a beginning it was! World War II was over. The world and the United States were at peace. Citizens were going to enjoy the "good life" and make sure their children had many of the opportunities and things they had not had during their early years. Prosperity was within reach of many. The "middle class" emerged as an identifiable segment of society. Home ownership was within reach, and having one's home became the symbol of the American dream. The economy flourished while it moved from war production to consumer-driven production. The good life came with a host of consumer products and devices to make life easier: television, improved radios, air conditioning, automatic dishwashers, freezers and refrigerators, and new automobiles. Bess Meyerson, June Cleaver, and Ozzie and Harriet were our role models. We felt good about ourselves in many ways. We were integrating sports[10] and had approved civil rights legislation.[11] We had proved that we could be the world's peacekeeper in Korea and had supported the creation of Israel.[12] We were creating a better world for our children! Life was close to perfect as exemplified by Don Larsen and his perfect World Series game in October 1956. Of course, we still had to go to work every day and that darn "rock and roll" music was everywhere.

During the preceding decade there had been some incidents that might have suggested to the acute observer that the American dream might not be all it seemed to be. But few, if any, would have imagined that the next twenty years would test both the validity of that dream and the values it represented.

Many Americans were shocked by the October 4, 1957, announcement that the Russians had launched an earth-orbiting satellite,[13] Sputnik, and this led to a major crisis of confidence. This challenge to America's scientific capabilities was only one of several events exploding into the headlines, onto TV screens, and forcing Americans to face some difficult questions about themselves.

The "rock" music movement[14] popularized by Alan Freed in Cleveland (1951) and peopled by the likes of Bill Haley, Jerry Lee Lewis, Chuck Berry, and Elvis Presley burst on the scene. Following closely behind was the "alienation" theme employed by movies featuring Marlon Brando and Jimmy Dean. Suddenly it was becoming popular to be a rebel, to join the "counterculture," and to live in "the Village." Long hair became popular (nothing seemed to aggravate parents more than long hair on their male children) and the term "beatnik" was coined to describe those who chose this lifestyle.[15]

The sexual revolution was also in full swing before the 1960s.[16] Kinsey's book on male sexual behavior was published in 1947 and caused an uproar along with much indignation. The decade leading up to the 1960 FDA approval[17] of Enovid E, the first oral contraceptive, was the decade of Margaret Sanger, who championed birth control and a woman's right to control her own body. The women's liberation movement was born. The 1956 publication of Grace Metalious's *Peyton Place,* with its feminist hero, added fuel to fires already burning.[18]

The civil rights movement also began prior to 1957. President Eisenhower signed into law civil rights legislation in the mid-1950s. The Supreme Court said no to "separate but equal" funding for education in 1954.[19] Rosa Parks took her famous bus ride on December 1, 1955.[20] Subsequent events in the fight for civil rights were seared into the nation's consciousness by TV, which brought us the agony and the hatred in real time. Martin Luther King emerged as the leader of this movement.

Politics and international relations were also producing some actions that would cause concern. The "Sputnik" space satellite was already mentioned. A hydrogen bomb was detonated on March 1, 1954.[21] Then we watched as the Russians got the "bomb." The CIA was instrumental in bringing the shah to power in Iran in 1953.[22] Our involvement in Vietnamese affairs escalated from just a few military advisors to the French military after Dien Bien Phu fell in May of 1954.[23] Much more noticeable to the average American was the fall of Cuba to Fidel Castro in early 1959[24] and the U-2 incident in which the Russians shot down an American spy plane.[25] The outrage of the McCarthy hearings had settled into an anticommunist attitude which was spurred on by these latter two events—one so close to home and the other bringing us face-to-face with the uncomfortable truth that our own country was in the spy business.

As the 1960s approached, the American dream was still alive, but self-doubt and an introspective mood had begun to permeate the public. The Kennedy presidency, in part, was a reaffirmation that the dream was still viable and achievable by many Americans. But events were to drive us deeper into self-doubt and serious concern for the safe passage of our country through those tumultuous times. The

1960 Kennedy/Nixon presidential campaign was a watershed event in America and in American politics. The power of television as an instrument of politics was firmly established. In that campaign, all the dreams, hopes, issues, and problems noted in the preceding paragraphs were politicized as never before. Politics encompassed all the issues and became a dominant influence in the fabric of American life. Special interest politics became the rule rather than the exception. Where would this lead us?

Tumultuous times and events gave even the most ardent patriot cause for introspection and questioning. Major events between 1962 and 1976 seemed to traumatize the public and provided few, if any, answers in a political climate seemingly driven to excess because of uncontrollable emotions about events and single interest issues. Events worthy of note included three political assassinations, an unpopular Asian war, a dramatic increase in recreational drug abuse/misuse, increased intensity by the civil rights movement and the women's liberation movement, "Watergate," a presidential resignation and pardon, and an Arabian oil embargo with its subsequent economic upheaval. And in spite of the swirling turmoil, there were positive developments, including the passage of legislation authorizing Medicare and Medicaid,[26] Americans walking on the moon, and the celebration of the 200th birthday of the nation.

CHANGES IN THE MEDICAL
AND PHARMACY WORLDS

At the same time the changes noted in the previous section were impacting the nation, the medical and pharmacy worlds were changing as well. Some changes were clearly the result of advances in technology and practice. Other changes occurred in response to national events, perceived needs of the public, and influences from outside of medicine and pharmacy.

Although often not as dramatic as the social and political changes occurring during this period, the advances in medicine and pharmacy were no less important for individual Americans. The single medical advance that can most closely be linked to a national event was the development and marketing of the anticonception medicines in the 1950s and 1960s. This advance clearly gave impetus to the sexual revolution and women's rights movements, and at least some of the funding for the basic research on these drug agents came from friends of those movements. Another pharmacologic leap forward was the development of antipsychotic medicines, including tranquilizers, that would help some to control the increasingly frantic pace of modern life. Other less direct linkages could be seen later in the period with national legislation focused on resolving one or more social issues requiring the health professions to participate in the proposed remediation.

In the medical world, the blossoming pharmaceutical industry began to develop and market amazing drug products.[27] In addition to the anticonception drugs and the impact they had, new antibiotics, including tetracycline, chloramphenicol, semisynthetic penicillins, and cephalosporins, were developed to fight infections. With the introduction of standardized *Rauwolfia serpentina* in 1953, the industry developed and made available chlorpromazine, meprobamate, prochlorpromazine, chlordiazepam, and diazepam. These drug agents revolutionized the management of psychoses by largely replacing convulsive shock therapy and surgery for treating patients with these conditions. Other major advances included diuretics, methyldopa, cortisone, propranolol, and polio vaccines.

The medical establishment continued to champion public health measures through the promotion of vaccination programs for children, including the newly available polio vaccines and the promotion of fluoridation of water supplies to assist in the development of strong teeth and the reduction of caries. The movement to enrich foodstuffs by adding vitamins and minerals as supplements continued. As the abuse and misuse of drugs, both legal and illicit, grew, the medical professions joined groups as diverse as the Food and Drug Administration and consumer interest groups in public campaigns. The objective was to make the public aware of the dangers inherent in the use of marijuana, LSD, cocaine, heroin, and other less well-known hallucinogens. There was a parallel objective to explain the dangers of misuse of prescription and nonprescription medications, including overdosing and underdosing, multiple prescriptions for the same class of products, taking someone else's medicine, and polypharmacy.

Advances in open-heart surgery and organ transplantation during these years provided hope to many. The medical profession itself continued its movement to specialization. The terms "health maintenance organization" and "managed care" appeared for the first time in American medicine as did Medicare and Medicaid. These latter legislative efforts were designed to provide access to medical care and the means to pay for it for aged and poor Americans. The passage of the Medicare and Medicaid legislation led to questions about the supply of health care manpower. The subsequent health professions manpower development grants provided many health profession schools with much needed capital for growth. The final major trend was the beginnings of accountability of the health care system to individuals and groups who were outside of the medical community—laymen.

The pharmacy world shared many of these noteworthy events for the medical world and had its unique events as well. We have already talked about the coming of age of the pharmaceutical industry. Other events in the educational, legal, and practice realms occurred to perplex and occupy pharmacy's attention during this period. In the educational realm, the thirty-year period from the Elliott Survey through the Millis Commission saw an extended debate on the virtues of the BS versus those of the PharmD degree. Much more will be said about this debate in the text that follows as it provided a major link between the Elliott study and the Millis Commission study. In brief, despite the Elliott study's recommendation that schools move from a four-year bachelor degree to a six-year program leading to the PharmD degree,[28] the AACP approved a compromise five-year curriculum leading to a BS in pharmacy degree to begin in 1960.[29] The additional year of study was to allow schools to revise their curricula to include more general education in the social sciences and incorporate the advances in the pharmaceutical sciences into the material presented to students. Two California schools (University of Southern California and University of California–San Francisco) moved to a six-year program in the mid-1950s while all the other schools went for the five-year program. In the mid-1960s the clinical pharmacy movement emerged and captured the attention of pharmacy educators. This movement focused on patient care, involvement of pharmacists as part of health care teams, and the provision of drug information to other health care professionals and patients. Other schools were keen on implementing clinical pharmacy programs, and they used grant dollars from the health professions' development moneys to get those programs started. Two other trends occurring during those years were noteworthy: Mandatory continuing education for practitioners started in 1967 in Kansas and Florida,[30] and the percentage of graduates that were women began to show sharp increases up from 10 percent in 1954 to 30 percent in 1976.[31]

On the legislative front, pharmacy was confronted with a number of new federal laws regulating various aspects of the pharmaceutical enterprise. On the state level, antisubstitution laws passed in the late 1940s began to be replaced with generic selection laws beginning in 1970.[32] In 1952, the Durham-Humphrey Amendments to the 1938 Food and Drug Act were passed.[33] Some professional decisions traditionally made by pharmacists were curtailed by that legislation, such as the requirement that pharmacists have a legitimate prescription before dispensing legend drugs and that prescribers indicate the number of refills they wanted for the specific prescription. The 1962 amendments[34] to the 1938 Food and Drug Act required that new drug products be proved effective as well as safe, required much more stringent controls on the investigational period of drug development, and imposed restrictions on advertising of prescription medications. Control of dangerous and addictive drugs was the goal of Congress's passage of the 1970 Comprehensive Drug Abuse Prevention and Control Act[35] and the Controlled Substances Act.[36] The latter created the Drug Enforcement Administration to coordinate enforcement efforts related to addictive and dangerous drugs.

Changes were made on the licensure and practice fronts as well. The National Association of Boards of Pharmacy (NABP) worked long and hard to develop and implement a national examination for candidates for licensure and finally offered the NABPLEX examination in the 1970s.[37] In practice, pharmacists endured the legal and regulatory requirements imposed on them and began the era of third-party prescription payment plans in the late 1960s.[38] Chain drugstore outlets continued to grow as did the numbers of pharmacists and prescriptions.[39] The number of pharmacists grew from 94,800 in 1947 to 119,500 in 1973. These pharmacists filled 371 million prescriptions worth $544 million in 1948 and 1,050 million prescriptions worth $4 billion in 1970 (not counting those prescriptions filled in hospitals, which would have raised the total to over 2 billion prescriptions). The per capita expenditure for drugs and drug sundries was $11.16 in 1950 and had grown to $39.91 in 1972. The impact on medical care of the pharmaceutical industry's prolific research, development, and promotion of drug products was clearly reflected in those numbers.

During the years 1946 to 1976 the profession reflected the changes in the general population. The hope and promise of immediately solidifying the image of the pharmacist as a health care professional after World War II did not materialize. The leadership of various segments of the profession got caught up in debate over which curricula should be followed. This resulted in the loss of some prerogatives through legislation and the issue of the role of pharmacy in health care remained unresolved. The pharmacist faced an increasing work load that focused on dispensing. There were continuing questions about how services and product should be valued and paid. The profession ushered in the post–World War II era with a national study of pharmacy and ended 1976 with the report of another national study of pharmacy. In the thirty-year period between those studies, the world in which pharmacists were educated and practiced changed almost completely. Those changes were reflected by the differences in approach and the results obtained by the respective studies.

DIFFERENT STUDIES FOR DIFFERENT TIMES

Our purpose was to examine the differences between the Elliott study and recommendations and the Millis Commission study and recommendations and to identify the bases for those differences if at all possible. We will get to that in this section. First, we should examine any studies about pharmacy that might have occurred between the Elliott and Millis studies to see if they can shed any light on differences that might appear from one end of a thirty-year period to the other end of that period.

There were nine studies conducted and another proposed during the thirty-year period between the two major reports under consideration[40] (Table 1.1). We did not consider *The Pharmaceutical Curriculum* a separate survey, as it was prepared from the materials on curriculum developed by the Elliott study but not published until 1952.[41]

The fact that so many different organizations, agencies, and individuals studied pharmacy suggests that there were serious questions about pharmacy and its professional status. And indeed, many of those studies, beginning with the 1965 paper by Sonnedecker on a proposed national study, considered the question of what professional roles were possible for pharmacists that would also be relevant to society and part of the medical care system.[42] In one sense, the

Millis Commission is a major effort to answer that question. Moreover, the question itself reflected that a different climate existed at the time of the Millis Commission study relative to the climate that existed immediately after World War II.

What were the differences in climate that existed in 1946 and in the early 1970s? In 1946, pharmacists still made many professional judgments in their day-to-day activities, including the selection of the drug product(s) and judgments about refilling prescriptions. The role of drug maker in the sense of compounding prescriptions still existed, although the extent of compounding was small and often involved mixing ingredients prepared by others. The public respected pharmacists and their efforts on behalf of their communities. There was little federal government involvement in health care. The focus of health care workers was on individual patients and the medical needs of those patients. In keeping with this climate, the Elliott study was an internal assessment of the profession with the goal of making the profession better. As Sonnedecker saw it, the study focused on "placing the needs of pharmacy education in relation to the status of other segments of American pharmacy at mid century."[43]

In contrast, the climate in the early 1970s was much different. The pharmacist's exercise of professional judgment had been decreased by legislation. He was still unable to select the source of drug products called for by his prescription. The amount of compounding the pharmacist did was minuscule in most practice sites. The public had begun to wonder what it was that he did behind the counter. The federal government had become very involved in health care, including redirecting the focus of care from the individual to society's needs as determined by legislators. The federal government also became a major purchaser of health care. Accountability to the federal government was suddenly in vogue. Society's health care needs were seen as equal in importance to the needs individuals might have. In keeping with this climate, the Millis Commission was an external study about moving the focus of pharmacy education to produce practitioners to meet the needs of society and the health care system.

Reflecting the different climates in which the studies were conducted, the foci and aims of the two studies were also different. The Elliott study aimed to "assemble . . . the critical facts relating to present day pharmaceutical education, practices, services and trade." These facts were to serve as the basis for "proposals designed for the

progressive betterment of pharmacy as a profession" with an emphasis on education as the vehicle for pursuing this betterment.[44] The
methodology used by the Elliott study included a survey of prescriptions, building on curriculum studies already completed, and a multi-
tude of surveys and interviews of pharmacy leaders, organizations,
and pharmacists.[45]

In contrast, the focus of the Millis Commission was stated in the
introduction to *Pharmacists for the Future.*

> It is against this background of deep and widespread concern
> about drugs, about pharmacy, and about pharmacists that the
> Study Commission on Pharmacy undertook its assignment to
> examine pharmacy education and to make recommendations
> designed to improve the education and training of pharmacists
> to the end that some of the drug-related problems may be solved
> and thereby the citizens of the nation may be better served.[46]

The Commission stated that it conceived of the health care delivery
system as a matrix, and continued, "The pharmacist is one of the elements of the matrix as he provides a drug-related service. . . . In this
matrix there are interfaces between the pharmacist and each of the
other individuals, institutions, and organizations"; the Commission
ended by indicating that it would "examine systematically many of
these interfaces by consulting with appropriate representatives of the
other elements of the matrix."[47] The methodology used by the Millis
Commission was due consideration of the current situation in health
care, the acknowledgment and appreciation of the role of the pharmaceutical industry and the government, and multiple consultations
with those individuals, organizations, and institutions that interacted
with pharmacists.[48] There was no survey of prescriptions conducted.
The impact of government involvement in health care and of society's
preoccupation with and trepidation about drug misuse can be clearly
seen in the focus of the Millis Commission's deliberations.

The recommendations of the two studies addressed pertinent issues for each in concert with the climate in which each study was
completed and in consideration of the focus of each study. Both studies addressed four similar issues: teachers, students, curriculum, and
degrees. However, the focus of the recommendations was different
for each study. We will consider these four issues more fully in the
text that follows. *The Pharmaceutical Survey* made multiple recom-

mendations for eleven issues.[49] Of the seven issues covered by the Elliott study and not covered by the Millis Commission, three issues focused on state boards of pharmacy[50] and generated a number of recommendations, including that the boards be separate state agencies to minimize political interference, that the boards develop a standard practice act, that the boards develop and use a national examination (achieved in the 1970s), that the boards' examination be based on practical aspects only, that the boards develop a more practical experiential prerequisite for candidates, and that the boards develop preceptors by means of visits and constructive reports to and from preceptors.

The Elliott Survey also made a number of recommendations to NABP regarding pharmacy manpower data[51] to the end that data should be collected systematically so that it would be available to whomever needed it. Recommendations about the American Council on Pharmaceutical Education (ACPE)[52] were related to recognition as the national accrediting agency in pharmacy, provision of support from constituent organizations, and implementation of a number of process improvements. Concerning finances[53] for pharmacy education, it was recommended that the schools and colleges advise their administrations of the financial needs and for the "businesses" of pharmacy to help support pharmacy education. Recommendations were made about the prescription survey data[54] specifically to base the curriculum, in part, on these data and to share these data among the schools of pharmacy. The last issue to receive recommendations was the subject of in-service training.[55] The recommendations of this issue involved the schools becoming responsible for providing in-service instruction, continuing education courses, and systematic visits to pharmacists in their areas, and encouraging state boards to create statewide organizational groups for such education.

For its part, the Millis Commission made a recommendation on one issue that was not considered by the Elliott study, namely, the creation of a national board of pharmacy examiners to credential pharmacists as specialists.[56] With this recommendation, it seems that the Millis Commission was responding to calls for specialty status by some in the profession. In 1976, it was not clear that a desire for specialty status would eventually lead to the American Pharmaceutical Association's (APhA) Board of Pharmaceutical Specialties and its processes for determining specialty designations. Given the Elliott study focus on improving education at large, it was understandable that no recommendations on specialization were forthcoming.

As noted, the four issues on which both studies made recommendations were teachers, students, curriculum, and degrees. The Elliott study recommended that the schools should try to balance the supply of teachers[57] with the demands of the curriculum; that salaries, teaching load, and research opportunities be adjusted to provide maximum support for all teachers; that the schools should offer in-service programs to help teachers learn new skills; that schools encourage teachers to pursue graduate studies; and that the American Foundation for Pharmaceutical Education (AFPE) fund fellowships for these teachers. All these recommendations were focused on helping schools develop faculty appropriate to their needs in the educational environment. In contrast, the Millis Commission recommended that schools provide appropriate practice opportunities for faculty having clinical teaching responsibilities and that schools train a modest number of *clinical scientists*.[58] The inference by the Millis Commission was that the schools had been successful in responding to the recommendations of the Elliott study and had been able to develop the additional faculty they needed to handle their educational programs in most areas. The Millis Commission wanted the schools to work as hard and as successfully to develop their clinical pharmacy faculty. The recommendation for training clinical scientists came from the conceptualization of health care delivery as a system in which pharmacy was a subsystem. The hope seemed to be that faculty expertise could be developed in the systemwide use of drug products and their application to every facet of patient care. These experts would be called clinical scientists. They would study the processes involved in moving a medicine from discovery through patient care and the system that used the processes.

The second issue covered by both studies was that of students.[59,60] The Elliott study made recommendations that promoted the matriculation of increasingly better students in the belief that better students would make better pharmacists. These recommendations included the use of standard IQ and aptitude entrance tests, providing guidance and counseling centers for students, and developing a handbook on opportunities in the profession to attract better students. The Millis Commission made no recommendations regarding undergraduate professional students and their recruitment. The Millis Commission did recommend that schools having the necessary resources should develop programs for graduate study and advanced professional education for more differentiated roles in practice. Of course, the recommendation about clinical scientists also applied to the recommendations about advanced/graduate study. That the Millis Commission was able to focus on advanced programs/graduate study in its recommendations strongly suggested that the schools of pharmacy had made great strides in improving their recruitment of better students for their first professional degree programs. As a result of this progress, the Millis Commission was able to make recommendations for additional educational programs that would move the profession forward.

The third issue which was addressed by both studies was that of curriculum. The Elliott study made recommendations[61] that were designed to strengthen the curricula of first professional degree programs including: improve student selection; improve dispensing prowess; improve study of how to administer a pharmacy; make students conscious of ethics; make students understand the need for cooperation with the other health professions; encourage students to participate in the activities of the profession; be sure that students are prepared to be responsible citizens with appropriate backgrounds in culture, values, and history; and improve and strengthen the pharmaceutical sciences already in the four-year curriculum.

The Millis Commission, in contrast, made recommendations[62] that appeared to encourage major changes in the curricula of the schools. Several recommendations stressed the need to focus the curricula on developing, organizing, and distributing *knowledge and information* about drugs with the idea that the pharmacist would provide drug information to consumers and health professionals as a major job component within a system of health care delivery. The Commission recommended that pharmacy be considered a "knowledge system in which *chemical substances and people called patients* interact" and that schools needed to "weigh physical/biological sciences versus the behavioral/social sciences in the curriculum." This seemed to suggest that schools needed to ensure that students were well-grounded in behavior and social science knowledge to ensure their capability to understand patients and their responses to drug therapy. The Millis Commission also recommended that the schools begin to provide an education that covered both a common body of knowledge, skills, attitudes, and behavior which all pharmacists must possess and "the differentiated and/or additional knowledge and skills required for specific practice roles."[63]

It was further recommended that schools base their curricula on competencies[64] which students should achieve rather than on the amount of knowledge available in any area of relevant science. While it might be difficult to determine exactly what the Millis Commission wanted schools to do relative to curricular content, it was clear that the members envisioned curricula much different than those based on the traditions of pharmacy in the twentieth century. The recommendation appeared to be curricula with less knowledge of science and more knowledge of patients and well people. The recommendations appeared to encourage differentiation of pharmacists while they were still students. And, finally, the recommendations suggested that the needs of society (in this instance, the need for knowledge about drugs and their actions in patients) become a major impetus for curricular change. What was clear in 1976 was that new ways of looking at curricula and determining curricular content were being offered to the profession for consideration and action.

The final issue that both studies made recommendations about was the entry-level degree in schools of pharmacy. The Elliott study recommended that schools adopt as soon as possible a six-year curriculum leading to a doctor of pharmacy degree as the first professional degree.[65] This recommendation was made in the belief that a two-plus four-year program would allow the schools to incorporate the advances in the pharmaceutical sciences as well as make sure that students had the general education courses that would promote good citizenship. The Millis Commission did not comment specifically on curriculum length or the degree designation that would be awarded for successful completion of the course of study. However, the Millis Commission appeared to base many of its recommendations on the assumption that most schools of pharmacy would offer a six-year program leading to the doctor of pharmacy degree. This assumption seemed particularly apparent with the recommendation[66] that a university health science center be considered the optimal environment for pharmacy education, with the understanding that alternative arrangement, if effectively utilized, could provide an acceptable environment for the education of students at the baccalaureate level. Of course, the issues of the six-year curriculum and the doctor of pharmacy degree as an entry-level degree for practice had not been resolved by 1976. Whether or not the assumptions inherent in the Millis Commission curriculum recommendations could work within the five-year BS curriculum (the minimum pharmacy education program) had not been determined.

SUMMARY COMMENTS

What kind of summary will suffice to tie together in some fashion all the distinctions noted in this chapter? We reviewed the Elliott study and found it to be an internally focused study about improving pharmacy education with the practice of pharmacy in existence in 1946. One would have to conclude that the Elliott study made appropriate and strong recommendations which led to the improvement of pharmacy education and to better practitioners during the period 1946 to 1976. Considering the changes occurring in the pharmacy world during that thirty-year period, including a "golden age" for the pharmaceutical industry and the many changes in legislation that impacted the profession, pharmacy education made remarkable strides in implementing the recommendations of the Elliott study and in strengthening the educational capabilities of the schools of pharmacy.

The very successes of the schools in creating strong educational programs paved the way for the Millis Commission recommendations that looked so different than those proposed by the Elliott study. And indeed, those recommendations were quite different. The Millis Commission appeared to assume that the schools were strong enough to handle recommendations calling for new ways to consider curricular development and would be able to incorporate expressions of society's health care needs into their curriculum development processes.

It was a thirty-year period filled with changes, many of which impacted pharmacy and pharmacy education. Change in pharmacy and in pharmacy education did not come as fast as some might have wished. However, change did come, following on the paths laid out by the Elliott study in many instances. The recommendations of the Elliott report identified specific tasks that needed to be done, who should do them, and, in some instances, how those tasks should be done. For the most part, those tasks were positive for the profession and its educational infrastructure. More important, the changes led to an environment in pharmacy and pharmacy education that fostered the Millis Commission and its recommendations for future growth of the profession and its educational programs. Because of the remarkable strides taken by pharmacy education in the intervening thirty years, the Millis Commission report recommendations identified what needed to be done without specifying who should do them or how they should be done. The Millis Commission report recognized that it could count on the "experts" in the colleges of pharmacy to address these needs in appropriate fashions. No stronger endorsement of the confidence and self-reliance of the colleges of pharmacy could have been made in 1975.

NOTES

1. A.E. Schwarting, "Address of the President: Some Propositions for Progress," *Am. J. Pharm. Educ.,* 36, 353 (1972).

2. *Pharmacists for the Future: The Report of the Study Commission on Pharmacy* (Health Administration Press, Ann Arbor, MI, 1975).

3. W. Skinner, "Summary of Selected Surveys and Conferences Concerning Pharmacy" (Unpublished manuscript, 42 pp.), University Archives, Case Western Reserve University, Classification # 1DD9, Box 43, Folder 1.

4. W.W. Charters, A.B. Lemon, and L. Monell, *Basic Material for a Pharmaceutical Curriculum* (McGraw-Hill Book Company, New York, 1927).

5. E.C. Elliott, *The General Report of the Pharmaceutical Survey, 1946-49* (American Council on Education, Washington, DC, 1950).

6. *Pharmacists for the Future: The Report of the Study Commission on Pharmacy* (Health Administration Press, Ann Arbor, MI, 1975), pp. 31-39 [pp. 167-171].*

7. *Pharmacists for the Future: The Report of the Study Commission on Pharmacy* (Health Administration Press, Ann Arbor, MI, 1975), p. 6 [p. 152].

8. E.C. Elliott, *The General Report of the Pharmaceutical Survey, 1946-49* (American Council on Education, Washington, DC, 1950), p. 3.

9. E.C. Elliott, *The General Report of the Pharmaceutical Survey, 1946-49* (American Council on Education, Washington, DC, 1950), p. 9.

10. D. Halberstam, *The Fifties* (Villard Books, New York, 1993), pp. 692-698.

11. T.H. White, *In Search of History* (Harper & Row, New York, 1978), p. 408.

12. M. Miller, *Plain Speaking: An Oral Biography of Harry S. Truman* (Berkley Publishing Corp., New York, 1973), pp. 213-218.

13. D. Halberstam, *The Fifties* (Villard Books, New York, 1993), pp. 624-625.

14. D. Halberstam, *The Fifties* (Villard Books, New York, 1993), pp. 456-473.

15. D. Halberstam, *The Fifties* (Villard Books, New York, 1993), pp. 295-307.

16. D. Halberstam, *The Fifties* (Villard Books, New York, 1993), pp. 272-281.

*Bracketed pagination refers to pages in Appendix A.

17. D.L. Cowen and W.H. Helfand, *Pharmacy: An Illustrated History* (Harry N. Abrams, Inc., Publishers, New York, 1990), pp. 194-206.

18. D. Halberstam, *The Fifties* (Villard Books, New York, 1993), pp. 577-578.

19. T.H. White, *In Search of History* (Harper & Row, New York, 1978), p. 373.

20. D. Halberstam, *The Fifties* (Villard Books, New York, 1993), pp. 539-563.

21. D. Halberstam, *The Fifties* (Villard Books, New York, 1993), p. 345.

22. D. Halberstam, *The Fifties* (Villard Books, New York, 1993), pp. 360-369.

23. T.H. White, *In Search of History* (Harper & Row, New York, 1978), p. 373.

24. D. Halberstam, *The Fifties* (Villard Books, New York, 1993), pp. 717-720.

25. D. Halberstam, *The Fifties* (Villard Books, New York, 1993), p. 710.

26. D.L. Cowen and W.H. Helfand, *Pharmacy: An Illustrated History* (Harry N. Abrams, Inc., Publishers, New York, 1990), p. 235.

27. D.L. Cowen and W.H. Helfand, *Pharmacy: An Illustrated History* (Harry N. Abrams, Inc., Publishers, New York, 1990), pp. 194-206.

28. E.C. Elliott, *The General Report of the Pharmaceutical Survey, 1946-49* (American Council on Education, Washington, DC, 1950), p. 230.

29. G.A. Sonnedecker, *Kremers and Urdang's History of Pharmacy,* 4th. Ed. (J. B. Lippincott Company, Philadelphia, 1976), pp. 240-241.

30. G.A. Sonnedecker, *Kremers and Urdang's History of Pharmacy,* 4th. Ed. (J. B. Lippincott Company, Philadelphia, 1976), p. 247.

31. D.L. Cowen and W.H. Helfand, *Pharmacy: An Illustrated History* (Harry N. Abrams, Inc., Publishers, New York, 1990), p. 236.

32. See Act No. 155, Laws of 1970, State of Michigan and other state pharmacy laws.

33. G.A. Sonnedecker, *Kremers and Urdang's History of Pharmacy,* 4th. Ed. (J. B. Lippincott Company, Philadelphia, 1976), p. 222.

34. G.A. Sonnedecker, *Kremers and Urdang's History of Pharmacy,* 4th. Ed. (J. B. Lippincott Company, Philadelphia, 1976), p. 222.

35. G.A. Sonnedecker, *Kremers and Urdang's History of Pharmacy,* 4th. Ed. (J. B. Lippincott Company, Philadelphia, 1976), p. 225.

36. G.A. Sonnedecker, *Kremers and Urdang's History of Pharmacy,* 4th. Ed. (J. B. Lippincott Company, Philadelphia, 1976), p. 530, note 49.

37. M.W. Green, *Epilogue, Prologue: From the Past Comes the Future* (National Association of Boards of Pharmacy, Chicago, 1979).

38. R.C. Johnson, private communication, January 18, 1983.

39. G.A. Sonnedecker, *Kremers and Urdang's History of Pharmacy,* 4th. Ed. (J. B. Lippincott Company, Philadelphia, 1976), pp. 299-313.

40. W. Skinner, "Summary of Selected Surveys and Conferences Concerning Pharmacy" (Unpublished manuscript, 42 pp.), University Archives, Case Western Reserve University, Classification # 1DD9, Box 43, Folder 1.

41. L.E. Blauch and G.L. Webster, *The Pharmaceutical Curriculum* (American Council on Education, Washington, DC, 1952).

42. G.A. Sonnedecker, "Exploratory Paper for a Proposed National Study of Pharmacy As a Professional Occupation" (Unpublished manuscript for the American Pharmaceutical Association, Washington, DC, 1965).

43. G.A. Sonnedecker, "Exploratory Paper for a Proposed National Study of Pharmacy As a Professional Occupation" (Unpublished manuscript for the American Pharmaceutical Association, Washington, DC, 1965), p. 253.

44. E.C. Elliott, *The General Report of the Pharmaceutical Survey, 1946-49* (American Council on Education, Washington, DC, 1950), p. 3.

45. E.C. Elliott, *The General Report of the Pharmaceutical Survey, 1946-49* (American Council on Education, Washington, DC, 1950), pp. 5-11.

46. *Pharmacists for the Future: The Report of the Study Commission on Pharmacy* (Health Administration Press, Ann Arbor, MI, 1975), p. 4 [p. 151].

47. *Pharmacists for the Future: The Report of the Study Commission on Pharmacy* (Health Administration Press, Ann Arbor, MI, 1975), p. 16 [p. 152].

48. *Pharmacists for the Future: The Report of the Study Commission on Pharmacy* (Health Administration Press, Ann Arbor, MI, 1975), p. x [pp. 147-148].

49. E.C. Elliott, *The General Report of the Pharmaceutical Survey, 1946-49* (American Council on Education, Washington, DC, 1950), pp. 210-232.

50. E.C. Elliott, *The General Report of the Pharmaceutical Survey, 1946-49* (American Council on Education, Washington, DC, 1950), pp. 220-224.

51. E.C. Elliott, *The General Report of the Pharmaceutical Survey, 1946-49* (American Council on Education, Washington, DC, 1950), pp. 210-213.

52 E.C. Elliott, *The General Report of the Pharmaceutical Survey, 1946-49* (American Council on Education, Washington, DC, 1950), pp. 213-216.

53. E.C. Elliott, *The General Report of the Pharmaceutical Survey, 1946-49* (American Council on Education, Washington, DC, 1950), pp. 225-226.

54. E.C. Elliott, *The General Report of the Pharmaceutical Survey, 1946-49* (American Council on Education, Washington, DC, 1950), pp. 226-228.

55. E.C. Elliott, *The General Report of the Pharmaceutical Survey, 1946-49* (American Council on Education, Washington, DC, 1950), pp. 230-232.

56. *Pharmacists for the Future: The Report of the Study Commission on Pharmacy* (Health Administration Press, Ann Arbor, MI, 1975), p. 143 [p. 237].

57. E.C. Elliott, *The General Report of the Pharmaceutical Survey, 1946-49* (American Council on Education, Washington, DC, 1950), pp. 216-218.

58. *Pharmacists for the Future: The Report of the Study Commission on Pharmacy* (Health Administration Press, Ann Arbor, MI, 1975), pp. 141-142 [p. 236].

59. E.C. Elliott, *The General Report of the Pharmaceutical Survey, 1946-49* (American Council on Education, Washington, DC, 1950), pp. 218-220.

60. *Pharmacists for the Future: The Report of the Study Commission on Pharmacy* (Health Administration Press, Ann Arbor, MI, 1975), p. 142 [pp. 236-237].

61. E.C. Elliott, *The General Report of the Pharmaceutical Survey, 1946-49* (American Council on Education, Washington, DC, 1950), pp. 229-230.

62. *Pharmacists for the Future: The Report of the Study Commission on Pharmacy* (Health Administration Press, Ann Arbor, MI, 1975), pp. 139-143 [p. 235].

63. *Pharmacists for the Future: The Report of the Study Commission on Pharmacy* (Health Administration Press, Ann Arbor, MI, 1975), p. 141 [p. 236].

64. *Pharmacists for the Future: The Report of the Study Commission on Pharmacy* (Health Administration Press, Ann Arbor, MI, 1975), p. 142 [p. 236].

65. E.C. Elliott, *The General Report of the Pharmaceutical Survey, 1946-49* (American Council on Education, Washington, DC, 1950), p. 230.

66. *Pharmacists for the Future: The Report of the Study Commission on Pharmacy* (Health Administration Press, Ann Arbor, MI, 1975), p. 143 [p. 237].

Chapter 2

Prelude to the Commission: The Intervening Years

Lawrence C. Weaver
Allen I. White
Dennis B. Worthen

INTRODUCTION

We were charged with the task of reviewing the intervening period between the time of the Pharmaceutical Survey and the Study Commission on Pharmacy. The events of these years provide insights into the creation of the Study Commission. The Pharmaceutical Survey was initiated in 1947 under the sponsorship of the American Council on Pharmaceutical Education. Dr. Edward C. Elliott, president emeritus of Purdue University, was chosen to be director of the survey. Under his dynamic leadership, and with the help of a staff of five assistants, a series of reports were published in 1948 and 1949 which became generally known as the "Elliott Report." The Study Commission on Pharmacy was developed under the sponsorship of the American Association of Colleges of Pharmacy in 1973. John S. Millis, chancellor emeritus of Case Western Reserve University and chairman of the National Fund for Medical Education, was named chair. The Study Commission became known as the "Millis Commission" and its final report, *Pharmacists for the Future,* was published in 1975. This chapter provides a synoptic review of activities during the period of 1948 to 1973 which, in our view, strongly influenced the creation of the Millis Commission.

The Elliott survey was undertaken in a time when the health care system was still adjusting to postwar changes. Pharmacists generally were inadequately prepared to meet the challenges created by the discovery, development, and marketing of new and more sophisticated medicines. They were also poorly prepared to deal with patients and other health professionals. In fact, during World War II, pharmacists were not commissioned as pharmacy officers since the military questioned whether pharmacy was a profession or a trade. The prewar "health team approach" to health care practiced by pharmacists and physicians was rapidly disappearing. Pharmacy reacted to these changes in diverse ways. We have selected developments which reflect the breadth and depth of the activities of the period. Truly, it was a time of change in pharmacy.

THE BEGINNING

The Pharmaceutical Survey (Elliott Report)

The nature and status of pharmacy practice in the United States had become a matter of concern to many of its leaders during the period between the two World Wars. Attempts to improve its professional standards were made, but without much success. The National Association of Boards of Pharmacy, the American Association of Colleges of Pharmacy, and the American Pharmaceutical Association were working together to promote a comprehensive survey of pharmacy as the basis for instituting changes to improve practice standards and the status of the profession of pharmacy. Economic conditions during the 1930s and the early 1940s and then World War II made it impossible to secure the funds to conduct such a survey. In 1945, the American Council on Education agreed to be the founding agency for the conduct of such a survey. With the financial support from the American Foundation for Pharmaceutical Education, the study began on April 15, 1946, under the title of the "Pharmaceutical Survey."

The use of the word "survey" in the title of the project gives definitive description to how the Elliott Commission was to undertake its task. The methodology, which was carried out by a group of experienced researchers, was to determine how pharmacy was practiced, what education was required to develop good practitioners, and to generally understand pharmacy and the world that pharmacy practiced in. The two overriding objectives were to assemble "the critical facts relating to present-day pharmaceutical education, practices, services and trade" and formulate "proposals designed for the progressive betterment of pharmacy as a profession—a profession steadily striving to have and to hold a distinctive place among the recognized health professions."[1]

The final report of the Elliott Commission collated the findings that had been gathered through the various surveys, including pharmacy organization, the education system and curriculum, and licensure and practice. The findings and recommendations were reported in eleven sections in Part XI of the General Report and approved by the Committee on the Pharmaceutical Survey. The sections are arranged in three parts—summary of the evidence, the problem, and recommendation. The recommendations are precise and focus on the purpose of the Pharmaceutical Survey, the formulation of programs of action for the advancement of pharmacy as a profession. Indeed, they were a significant part of the platform from which the advances in pharmacy were launched during the next several decades.

All of the findings and recommendations of the Pharmaceutical Survey were of interest and importance to pharmacy education. The sections could be broadly grouped as being practice, regulatory, or education focused (Table 2.1).

Practice Focused

Section 1 focused on the manpower requirements for trained professionals and concluded that there were no reliable data on the total number of licensed pharmacists or how they were employed. In addition, other demographics such as age and domicile were lacking. These deficits resulted in a lack of knowledge of how many pharmacists were truly needed to balance the supply and demand for trained professionals. Section 9 was an extensive prescription study that sought to understand what pharmacists, mostly in retail, did in order to fill a prescription. The finding was that almost 75 percent of all prescriptions dispensed were manufacturer specialties and required little manipulation other than affixing a label. This finding suggested that pharmacists were being trained, even at that time, for a function that comprised a small part of the duties in the pharmacy, extemporaneous compounding.

TABLE 2.1. The Pharmaceutical Survey

Part XI: Findings and Recommendations

Section	Focus	Title
Section 1	Practice	The Supply of, and the Demand for, Trained Pharmacists—Professional Manpower Records
Section 2	Education	The American Council on Pharmaceutical Education
Section 3	Education	The Teaching Staffs
Section 4	Education	Student Selection, Guidance and Testing
Section 5	Regulation	State Boards of Pharmacy: Organization, Financial Support, and Functions
Section 6	Regulation	State Boards of Pharmacy: Examinations for Licensure
Section 7	Regulation	State Boards of Pharmacy: Practical Experience Requirement for Licensure
Section 8	Education	The Financing of Pharmaceutical Education
Section 9	Practice	The Prescription Study
Section 10	Education	The Pharmaceutical Curriculum
Section 11	Education	In-Service Training for Pharmacists

Regulation Focused

Three sections, 5, 6, and 7, provided information about the status and activities of state boards of pharmacy. Since the state boards regulate entrance to the profession through the licensing exam and regulate minimum standards of practice, these sections were of great interest and importance to pharmacy education. Section 6 reported the review by education experts who questioned the relativity, validity, and reliability of the examination questions. A second series of questions were surveyed by experienced pharmacy educators to determine whether the examinations met the central objective of protecting public health and safety by assuring competent practitioners. Less than 40 percent of the questions were judged to be valid. Section 7 reported the then current status of practical experience required for licensure. The findings documented the role of practical experience in licensure but recommended that the experience be more professional (rather than clerical), task related and standardized, or abolished.

Education Focused

Section 2, concerning the American Council on Pharmaceutical Education (ACPE), was arguably the single most important section for pharmacy education. ACPE was charged with the establishment and application of educational standards. The standards would of necessity influence education in every aspect of operation and would even determine whether a school would exist. The Survey recommendations led to a strengthening of ACPE's ability to carry out its responsibilities.

Section 3, The Teaching Staffs, surveyed the availability of educators and their qualifications. The findings were both frank and alarming when pharmacy was compared to other professional education. The need for qualified teachers was increasing rapidly with expanding programs. Too many part-timers and those with a master's degree or less (approximately 45 percent of the faculties) were being employed. Low salaries were identified as a factor in education's inability to compete with industry for individuals with superior ability.

Section 4, Student Selection, Guidance and Testing, starts with the observation that competent students and competent teaching result in a competent profession. The Survey compared the scholastic ability of students entering pharmacy school with those entering other baccalaureate programs. An observation, perhaps prescient, was that screening for admission to pharmacy education was not comparable to medicine, law, or dentistry, because these professions had a two-year college study prerequisite.

Section 8, The Financing of Pharmaceutical Education, concludes that some schools are underfunded and may not be able to maintain necessary high standards. Interestingly, the solution recommended was that industry should be responsible for making up the shortfall and underwriting financial support of the schools. The basis for the recommendation was that medical schools were receiving more grants than pharmacy schools.

Section 10, The Pharmaceutical Curriculum, drew the most attention and was to have the greatest long-range impact. The two elements of the section that were to have the most lasting impact were the curriculum study and the recommendation for the establishment of a six-year degree. The Survey committee acknowledged that a critical examination and evaluation of the material and methods of instruction for preparing pharmacists for professional practice was a principal task of the Survey. It added:

> It was well known that this was a complicated and difficult undertaking. At no other point has there been more discussion and sharper differences of judgment among the profession. The issues involve what should be taught, how much, when, and to whom.
>
> When account is taken of the historical development of the program of pharmaceutical teaching, one cannot fail to be impressed by the tendencies to hold fast to the past. Adjustments of the schemes of instruction to changed and changing conditions have taken place slowly, but the old concepts, the old methods, and the old textbooks have continued to exercise a strong influence.[2]

The recommendations of the Survey were broad in scope and called for changes in the objectives of pharmaceutical education. Among its specific recommendations were the following:

1. . . . .
   F. Qualifying students to cooperate with members of the other health professions and to consult with them; to furnish accurate, objective, and scientific information to physicians and members of other health professions concerning drugs and their action.
   G. Preparing students to provide professional services to the public appropriate to the basic functions of pharmacy in its role as a health profession.
2. Continue their efforts for the constructive betterment of the existing four-year program of education and training providing the essential knowledge and skills for the practice of pharmacy leading to the degree of Bachelor of Science in Pharmacy.
3. Take the necessary initial steps for the development and establishment of a six-year program of education and training leading to the professional degree of Doctor of Pharmacy (Phar.D.), this

program to include two or more years of general education and basic science training.

4. Continue cooperative relationship of the Survey and the Committee on Curriculum of the American Association of Colleges of Pharmacy for the purpose of: (a) improving the four-year program, and (b) developing a six-year program; and that in these two undertakings, attention be given to the reports prepared by the Survey on instruction in pharmacognosy, pharmacy, physical sciences and mathematics, pharmacology and related sciences, microbiology and public health, and pharmacy administration.

5. Propose a plan whereby graduates in pharmacy who receive other degrees in this field become eligible for Candidacy for the degree Doctor of Pharmacy.[3]

Section 11, "In-Service Training for Pharmacists," dealt with the topic now called continuing education. At the time of the Elliott Report, interest in continuing education programs in the health professions was just beginning to develop. The rapid expansion of scientific knowledge and applications to the health professions led to the recognition of the need to provide continuing education. This would allow those whose formal education was not sufficient, or outdated, to meet the needs of contemporary practice and achieve the competency necessary to meet standards at the time of relicensure.

The Teachers Seminars

The Teachers Seminars were a direct result of Elliott's recommendation in Section 7 of the Survey Report. It was noted that there was a need to improve the quality of the faculties of the colleges of pharmacy if a number of the recommendations of the Survey were to be accomplished. To assist in accomplishing that goal, it was recommended that an annual summer seminar be established. The primary purpose was to provide an environment for educators and graduate students to share in formation of the "progressive content and methods of pharmaceutical teaching."[4]

There were two objectives identified for the first Teachers Seminar, which was held in 1949 at the University of Wisconsin.

> First, to present and make clear to teachers of pharmacy the
> newer facts and concepts concerning subject matter to be in-
> cluded in the area of pharmacy and, second, to arrange this sub-
> ject matter in organized courses in the curriculum to assure a
> logical presentation in the colleges.[5]

Among the papers presented were recommendations for the development and introduction of two new courses, physical pharmacy and
pharmacy technology. The concepts in those two courses marked the
beginning of an educational revolution in pharmacy. Traditional descriptive pharmacy courses were replaced by the scientifically based
courses which became pharmaceutics, biopharmaceutics, and pharmacokinetics.

The Pharmaceutical Curriculum

The *Pharmaceutical Curriculum* was the direct descendent of the
Pharmaceutical Syllabus, which was published several times between 1910 and 1945 with the objective of standardizing the curricula
in the pharmacy schools. Technically, however, the *Pharmaceutical
Curriculum* was part of Elliott's *Pharmaceutical Survey* although it
was not published until 1953 and was authored by Lloyd Blauch and
George Webster. The reason given for the delayed publication was to
prepare a more extensive report on the pharmaceutical curriculum.
Because of this delay, elements from the first few Teachers Seminars
were available for incorporation into the recommendations. The
study acknowledged the questions and problems that pharmaceutical
educators were facing. The issues ranged from the question of what
the education should be to prepare pharmacists for the practice of
pharmacy to what role pharmacy associations should play in the
development of the curriculum.

The conclusions were extremely candid. The lack of curriculum
balance and consistency was a concern. There was serious doubt that
all of the necessary subjects could be covered adequately in a four-
year program:

> None of the four-year programs include all of the instruction
> which, upon the advice of consultative committees, should be
> offered. The principle lacks are in general education, pharma-
> cology and allied sciences, and the administrative aspects of

pharmacy. The subject of pharmacognosy needs modernization and revision of its content. Physical chemistry and biochemistry have assumed an importance in modern medication which warrants increased attention to these subjects.[6]

It was clear that the four-year program was already fully loaded and there was need to add new courses. Of course, there was also the challenge to renew or remove items of diminishing relevance. The major point of controversy that developed was what the length and configuration of the period of study should be, 1-4, 2-3, or 2-4 years. The usual way to differentiate pharmacy programs is 1-4, 2-3, and so forth. It designates the number of years in the preprofessional stage and the number in the professional. The basis for the differences in selecting program length was positioned as follows:

The disagreement stems from two different views of the problem. One seeks to answer the question: what can be done which will improve the general quality and quantity of instruction in the colleges of pharmacy as they are now operating on a minimum four-year-after-high-school curriculum? The other poses the problem as: what quality and quantity of instruction is necessary to provide the pharmacist with the fundamentals of a professional education as outlined by the Committee on the Pharmaceutical Survey?[7]

THE INTERVENING YEARS

The Challenge to Pharmacy in Times of Change

In 1964 the American Pharmaceutical Association (APhA) and the American Society of Hospital Pharmacists (ASHP) cosponsored the Commission on Pharmacy Services to Ambulant Patients by Hospitals and Related Facilities. The Commission had thirteen members and, in addition to representatives of the APhA and the ASHP, included representatives of the American Hospital Association and the American Medical Association. The rationale for the establishment of the Commission was the shift in pharmaceutical services that were being provided in institutions, frequently for ambulatory patients, and the broader impact that this shift could or would have. The Commission had an overall objective of studying and understanding contemporary pharmacy practice which included the specific objective of learning about changes in pharmacy education, especially those that might be required because of the changing patterns in medical care and hospital utilization.

> In short, the profession needed to know what was going on within itself, whether the effect from the increase in pharmaceutical service to outpatients by hospitals might be weakening or strengthening the profession. The profession needed guidelines; it needed information about itself and the professional and social world of which it is a part.[8]

The Commission engaged Donald Brodie, a professor at the University of California–San Francisco College of Pharmacy, as a consultant. While Dr. Brodie was not charged with a specific assignment, he did undertake a study to understand the relationship between pharmacists and hospital practice. The results were to provide guidelines that might be useful to the profession. During the study, Brodie met with seventy-seven individuals to gain their perspectives. This group was largely composed of individuals involved in hospital administration (thirty-eight people) and pharmacy administration (twenty-four people). The remainder were physicians, individuals from the pharmaceutical industry, and other miscellaneous groups. The study report, *The Challenge to Pharmacy in Times of Change,* was completed and published in 1966. Chapter VI of the report focused on "Pharmacists and Pharmaceutical Services" and addressed components of practice, science, education, the pharmacist, and, finally, public concerns. In a relatively short thirteen pages Brodie identified a number of key concerns and recommended actions that included the profession in all settings, not just institutional.

Pharmacy Practice

In this section Brodie identified the dichotomous nature of retail pharmacy to be the underlying problem as pharmacists focused more on the mass distribution of convenience goods totally unrelated to health. The question truly became one of "what is pharmacy" since the function of creating medicines passed from the individual compounder to the manufacturer. Using the examples of the learned professions of theology, medicine, and law, Brodie raised the question of what the mainstream of pharmacy was, given the focus of the practitioner on nonprofessional activities and relegating the professional service of the public to a part-time basis.

> With the transfer of the scene of the development and production of drug products from the setting of the local pharmacy to that of the industry has come a decrease in the creative and an increase in the distributive responsibilities of the pharmacist. The pharmacist and the public alike have focused so much attention on the physical aspects of the distribution of a commodity that each has lost sight of the service that the pharmacist provides and the protection that his expertise assures the public.[9]

Brodie went forward to suggest that the ultimate goal of the profession must be the safe use of drugs by the public and that this function could best be identified as "drug-use control." Drug-use control was defined as "the sum total of knowledge, understanding, judgments, procedures, skills, controls, and ethics that assures optimal safety in the distribution and use of medication." He argued that drug-use control "provides a purpose, gives a direction, recognizes need and fulfillment in the patient-pharmacist relationship, and it is that basic ingredient which underlies the essentiality of pharmacy and its service."[10]

Pharmaceutical Science

Brodie identified that pharmacy had a role in both the creation of medical breakthroughs as well as the application of these breakthroughs into benefits for the individual patient. Pharmacy's role was put into three categories. The first was to work with other scientists to develop new knowledge that could be applied to new therapeutic areas. The second was to better understand and work to apply these new areas of knowledge to meet regulatory requirements. The third was to distribute the products through the network of outlets. While seemingly better placed in another section, he used the third category to state that the unifying function of the profession was to get the right drug to the right patient at the right time.

The final link in the distributive function results in closing the physician-patient-pharmacist triad: the pharmacist ultimately making the medication available to the patient. Regrettably, many pharmacy practitioners have minimized the importance of this direct confrontation with the patient by entrusting the responsibility to others. Pharmacists will find, as others have, that their greatest professional strength resides in the sincerity, integrity, and permanence of the pharmacist-patient bond. . . . His success will reflect the degree to which he fulfills these needs and the excellence of his service.[11]

Pharmaceutical Education

Brodie reviewed the education of various professions and the evolution of all of the major professions, except pharmacy, to the professional doctorate. The insight that emerged was that pharmacy education was influenced by a different force than the profession of medicine.

Pharmacy, because of its scientific make-up and the existing level of knowledge, inclined heavily to the physical sciences. Whether by design or not, it followed the educational leadership of chemistry and others, ignoring the fact that pharmacy is not a basic discipline, but one of applied sciences.[12]

Brodie continues this examination to review the recommendation that had emerged from the Elliott Survey for the creation of a six-year program leading to the PharmD degree. Clearly, the adoption of such a degree would have been an opportunity to place the professional education of the pharmacist on similar footing with other professional education programs. Instead, a compromise was reached in the late 1950s to continue the baccalaureate degree but expand the curriculum to a five-year program in 1960. Brodie took the position that despite any justification that might be offered in behalf of the profession at that time, the fact remains that the five-year curriculum was a compromise. To compromise professional education is to compromise the profession of which it is a part.[13]

The Pharmacist

While pharmacists have a long history of serving the public, there is a distinct change in practice. Pharmacy has become a more important part of the hospital and pharmacists have gained stature because of the knowledge and expertise that is provided to the institution. On the other hand, community pharmacy has moved away from the professional aspects of the profession and become more of a business, just like any other business. This has set up a problem as the public views the provision of a health service in a commercial setting that is largely devoted to non–health care products. Brodie is very forward in his view of this situation: "Pharmacists who work in these establishments on an employed basis often fail to maintain a professional identity within themselves. As a result they become leeches of the profession and contribute little to its welfare that is not self-centered."[14] In contrast, he points out the beginnings of a new practice model, pharmaceutical service. The pharmaceutical service center is seen as providing all of the services required for the provision of prescription services. Interestingly, this model also provides for complete patient profiles and other information devices that can be used by the patient and the physician. The dilemma is which model the practitioner will follow.

> He often is tempted to live a dual life—one as a professional, the other as a merchant. His only permanent worth to the community, however, lies in the services for which he alone is trained to provide. This worth can reach new heights in the years immediately ahead if he can see the new opportunity that awaits him because of the demand for his service and the knowledge he possesses. The pharmacist has reached the time when he can divest himself of many of the frustrations of his dilemma, if he will but do so.[15]

Summary and Recommendations

The summary and recommendations addressed the issues of the changing environment that pharmacy was developing within. In large part, the changes within the hospital and institutional setting were the focus of the summary, largely because of the original charge of the full Commission. However, two sections of the summary, Pharmaceutical

Education and Pharmacy's Stewardship, picked up the broader thread of professional need and reason for existence. It is in these two sections that there is an evident link between the Elliott Survey and the Millis Commission.

Pharmaceutical Education: As more medical care becomes institution based, and more pharmaceutical service is provided from an institutional environment, pharmacists with both knowledge of and training in institutional pharmacy will be required. The pharmacy curriculum, as the curriculum of other health professions, should be studied, with particular attention devoted to social sciences relating to health, biological sciences, and health institution administration.

Pharmacy's Stewardship: Contemporary social change has brought all professions to a time of self-examination. Pharmacy is called to a higher level of professional stewardship than it has known in the past, one that will require adaptation to a new code of socio-economic responsibility by all health professions. If the service of pharmacy to society continues to be dominated by its distributive function of which it has become a captive, it cannot fulfill the needs of a new social order. Only when pharmacy's contribution to society is dominated by the capacity of its practitioners to apply their scientific knowledge to the needs of society and by their concern for public health and safety will the profession be justified in claiming all of the privileges of an essential health service.[16]

Pharmacy-Medicine-Nursing Conference on Health Education

In honor of the university's sesquicentennial in 1967, the University of Michigan College of Pharmacy hosted a multidisciplinary conference that brought together the health professions of medicine, nursing, and pharmacy. This conference was a milestone event in the fact that it engaged medicine and nursing in the expanding question of what the new roles for pharmacy and pharmacists might be and how the health professions would have to cooperate to deliver the required improvements and increases of health care.

The first segment of the conference was devoted to three papers with a common title—"Emerging Patterns of Education and Practice in the Health Professions"—followed by the profession, that is, Medicine, Nursing, or Pharmacy. While different, each of the speakers noted the need to judge the health professions not on historical boundaries and prerogatives, but rather on the ability of the profession to directly enhance the health of people.

Dr. Brodie served as the presenter of the pharmacy portion of the program and addressed four broad topics: the medical-social revolution of the twentieth century, pharmacy and that revolution, practice changes, and emerging patterns in pharmacy education.

In his comments relating to the revolution, Brodie articulated that the changes in health care were driving changes in the health professions. In response, he believed that the entire role of pharmacy needed to be reexamined and defined. He challenged whether the drugstore was the place for pharmacists to practice and offered as the alternative what he called "modern pharmaceutical service." The need, as he saw it, was to get the pharmacist into a professional practice setting that would identify him as an expert both to other professions and to the public. In order to accomplish this, the patient would have to emerge as the central focus of education. He acknowledged that this would not be easy, and also identified the consequences of not trying.

> Notwithstanding the multiplicity of problems that the next twenty-five to thirty years hold for us, the profession of pharmacy, without doubt, will be called to a higher level of professional practice than it has known in the past. The years of transition will be difficult, and at times progress will be agonizingly slow. The status quo will not be maintained, and the alternatives seem clear: either the profession will rise to the new level of service to which it is called and its practitioners will become fully competent to become participating specialists on the health care team or the profession will regress and its members become technicians, trained by a correspondingly appropriate educational program.[17]

> We have an opportunity to take a high road, thereby achieving a new level of practice, and to develop education and training programs that will permit us to attain this level. It will be a long,

hard pull. If we choose the lower road, we will find a little easier pathway, perhaps, than if we choose the higher one, if for no other reason than it will be downhill. At this level of practice, we will have been reduced to an admitted level of technical performance with a corresponding educational preparation.[18]

The issue of educational relevance was a common theme for much of this conference. The point was that the educational program was the mechanism to prepare the professional for the role that he would fulfill in practice. The practice of medicine was clinical and so, therefore, was the educational program. Nursing was similarly oriented to patient care and education. Pharmacists, alone of all of the health professionals, were not trained with direct patient contact (that is, clinically) but focused on a product. While physicians and other health professionals were paid for providing a service, pharmacists practiced in a mercantile setting that suggested a conflict of interest between the need to sell something and the need of the patient. The question of what pharmacists were being educated for was also raised:

> The courses in pharmaceutical sciences, unfolding so rapidly as effective and worthy specializations of their own, as they are taught to undergraduate professional students tend to be focused upon the needs of the specialist in these sciences rather than upon the needs of the general practitioner. In many cases, the professional goal of a majority of the students goes unrecognized. In other cases, it is even ignored.[19]

At the conclusion of the conference, nineteen recommendations, in three broad categories, were summarized. Among the recommendations in each category were the following:

Role of the pharmacist:
5. The terms consultation or consultant (as applied to the pharmacist in relation to drugs) be clearly defined as used with reference to the laity as well as with reference to other health professionals.

Relationships among health professionals:
8. Continuous recognition of the health needs of the public be considered basic in revising or devising roles for the pharmacist

as well as for the nurse, the physician, and other health professionals.

Educational program:
14. The roles of the pharmacist of the future be anticipated as fully as is possible prior to any revolutionary revision of the pharmacy curriculum, recognizing that such anticipation can not be complete and that the pharmacist must serve in cooperation with other health professionals. This recommendation must not be thought of as discouraging innovation and experiment.[20]

Professional Pharmacy Seminar

In 1969, Eli Lilly held its third Professional Pharmacy Seminar and hosted faculty and deans representing seventy-five schools and colleges of pharmacy in the United States, Puerto Rico, and Canada. There were two objectives established for the three-day session. The first objective was to provide exposure in several scientific fields that might be of help to the schools in their efforts to redesign their curricula. Drug metabolism, toxicology, and clinical pharmacology were specially noted for their relevance to clinical pharmacy. The second objective, acknowledged as self-serving, was to expose academics to the personnel needs of Lilly in their future recruiting efforts. Even in the opening remarks, there was attention placed on the emergence of clinical pharmacy and the fact that it was an example of how the schools were working to upgrade their curricula. Clinical pharmacy was also identified as a "new area of truly professional service to prescription patrons. If our pharmacists assume this responsibility, and I am sure they will, their image as sellers of goods will be altered significantly."[21]

Henry DeBoest, vice president of Corporate Affairs for Lilly and later a member of the Millis Commission, noted that no one has any assurance of participating in the future by divine right, but must earn that privilege. The environment is changing at an increasing pace, and one of the changes is the public perspective of health care and the way that it is delivered. There is serious question whether the current health care system is meeting the needs of the people whom it is supposed to serve. The ability to meet the needs of people will be an essential measure of how health care professionals will be regarded in the future.

I believe that we must look not merely at what is good for pharmacy, what is good for the pharmaceutical industry, and what is going to advance the profession but at what is good for the public and what will meet the public's needs. This must become a primary consideration, because, ultimately, this will be the criterion by which we will either continue to exist or disappear. To satisfy this criterion may require quite a metamorphosis; but it is the ability to serve the public in a manner the public needs and wishes to be served that will determine the future existence of the various elements of the health-care team.[22]

The seminar was concluded with presentations from the visiting academics. Jack Orr, executive chairman of the American Association of Colleges of Pharmacy, recognized the need for educators to plan for the future. He stressed the difficulty of the task since there is no way to know what the practitioner of the future will be and that understanding is essential in determining what the curricula will need to be. He also noted that AACP was preparing a grant application to study the future of pharmacy education. Dr. Orr also recruited several new deans to provide a perspective on the future of pharmacy education.

Lawrence C. Weaver of the University of Minnesota looked to the future and suggested that there would be at least eight factors that would influence community pharmacy in the future. These factors ranged from the establishment of regional health care centers and their locations, the use of technology and ancillary personnel, and the payment system for prescriptions. One of his factors addressed the interplay between medicines and the public.

Drugs are being used, misused, and abused in unprecedented quantities and with unprecedented sophistication. Self-medication practices by the public are growing. How many patients have drug profile records that are properly used? Who consults with them on prescription and nonprescription products?[23]

Weaver also emphasized that education must lead practice through a curriculum that is responsive to the needs of the health care system. These needs will directly affect what is taught and how long it will take to teach it. He also acknowledged the need to have the education process be patient oriented as well as product oriented.

Raymond E. Hopponen of South Dakota State challenged the state of education by noting that it had led to the oft-heard axiom describing pharmacists as the most overeducated and underutilized health professional. The science and practice of pharmacy had become disassociated; what was being taught was not what was needed to practice. The pharmacist was disappearing from the public's eye and there was not a clear understanding of what the pharmacist did that was of value, other than moving pills from a big bottle to a little one. The result of this increasing dilemma was the evolving development of clinical pharmacy. Evolving is the correct word because of the many different ways that it was approached in the schools. Important issues such as the need to draw practitioners into the faculty to teach clinical skills and the need for training sites, whether they be medical centers, hospitals, or other areas where there is a potential for patient interaction, still needed to be addressed to determine the right way to proceed. AACP defined clinical pharmacy as

> that area within the pharmacy curriculum which deals with patient care with an emphasis on drug therapy. Clinical pharmacy seeks to develop a patient-oriented attitude [and that's probably the key to most of this—the patient-oriented attitude]. The acquisition of new knowledge is secondary to the attainment of skills in interprofessional and patient communications.[24]

Hopponen concluded his remarks by drawing the audience back to the essential point:

> clinical pharmacy, in my mind, is a concept and not just a course of instruction. We should create in the student an awareness of the patient as the recipient of medical care and develop in him an ability to communicate drug information to the patient and to the practitioner.[25]

Challenges to Pharmacy in the 1970s

In 1970, the National Center for Health Services Research and Development and the School of Pharmacy at the University of California–San Francisco hosted an invitational conference on pharmacy manpower. This conference focused on the relationship between pharmacists and physicians but included representatives of the other health care professions as participants. While there were several objectives for the conference stated, they can be summarized into one: "To examine critically emerging possible future roles for pharmacists in a system of comprehensive health care."[26]

In this broad ranging exchange a number of important points were emphasized by the participants, frequently from different perspectives. First, there was a general agreement that the shift in health care would continue to move from a one-person show to one that was more institutionalized. This did not mean that practice would necessarily be in a hospital. It did mean that there was a recognition of the need to structure the different providers into an organization that focused on delivering a total care package for the patient.

The discussion and debate between many of the participants included the establishment of the health care team and the need for a captain of the team, presumably the physician. Some challenged whether this would be the model for the future. Instead, they suggested that the first order of business would be to determine what needed to be done, what skills were required, and only then determine who should do what. The need for the future may be very different than what it was in the past and it was critical that old prerogatives, turf, and labels not dictate the future just because of history. This discussion was even further broadened by Vernon Wilson, the head of the Health Services and Mental Health Administration, Department of Health, Education and Welfare.

> Interdisciplinary conferences like this one are a relatively new phenomenon in the world of health. From time immemorial, like the legendary Lowells and Cabots, physicians have talked only with physicians, pharmacists with pharmacists, dentists with dentists. Only recently, impelled by the gradual recognition that no profession can reasonably subsist as an island, have we begun to pool our knowledge and share our problems. This is a healthy sign. Thus far, however, it seems to me that our interdisciplinary conferences have suffered from two shortcomings. First, their products have tended to be abundantly predictable. Each one calls for the creation and promulgation of the "health team," or the "teamwork approach to health." By contrast with the volume of lip service paid to this important concept, it is still very difficult to find a real health team in action outside of the institutional setting. Second, I would suggest that one very im-

portant participant in the health care process is being left out. He is not invited to our interdisciplinary deliverations, nor is he given due consideration in the health team concept. I refer, of course, to the patient.[27]

The question of the role of the pharmacist in the future emerged as the central theme. It was clear that the old role of the merchant who only spent part of the time in professional activities would not be sufficient to gain an influential role in the eventual team. This suggested that the question of what the pharmacist wouldn't do would be as important as deciding what he would do.

> The trend is toward the pharmacist being less and less available for personal consultation. The economics of pharmacy practice are moving him further and further away from the very people who have a greater and greater need for his help. Our efforts to make the pharmacist more qualified to function in this capacity will go for naught unless we find a way to reverse the trend of isolating the pharmacist from the people he should serve.[28]

A number of roles were suggested by the various participants. While the traditional activities of procuring, storing, and distributing medicines were acknowledged both for traditional excellence and need, it was clear that this might not be the role of a professional in the future. Drug information was an area of interest but the most energy focused on clinical pharmacy. However, even this suggestion was not without difficulties. For example, the question of how to educate or train clinical pharmacists presented some dilemma. In at least some situations, schools were simply adding the word "clinical" to old courses without changing content. This was due, in part, to a general understanding of what clinical pharmacy really was.

> Little thought has been given to the kind of roles to be played. You can talk all you want about subject matter content. You can talk all you want about curriculum, but it is irrelevant unless you consider the kinds of individuals you want to produce and what it is they are going to be doing in the profession. You have spent, I think, a small amount of time in first defining roles, and an inordinate amount of time is spent on curriculum and subject matter content. Very often it is a series of manipulations of courses,

their arrangement and adding adjectives or something else to describe the courses which really, in many cases, do not reflect the kind of role you expect the individual to play when he is a graduate of the profession . . . because so much time is spent on curriculum content, the curriculum tends to be designed in a vacuum. That is, not only is it unrelated to the role to be played by the pharmacist but unrelated to other health professions. . . . I question whether even the clinical pharmacist that we are now producing is realistic because, again, have we really defined the role of this particular individual? Furthermore, have we related this individual to other professions? . . . The trouble with curricula in the health professions is that they are like college catalogs; they continuously get larger, never smaller.[29]

Another possible role for the pharmacist was proffered by Henry Simmons, head of the Food and Drug Administration's Bureau of Drugs. In his presentation, he outlined the issue of the increasing misuse of drugs as a major societal problem. He was not referring to the use of illegal substances but rather the misuse and abuse of legitimate medicines. At that time the incidence of complications due to drug therapy was estimated to be 10 percent, and 5 percent of hospital admissions were due to serious drug reactions. This figured out to be approximately 1.5 million hospital admissions per year.

We have a major problem of drug misuse in this country. The efforts of all will be needed to correct it. I feel that the pharmacy profession, if properly utilized, can be a significant factor in its solution, in the solution of this health care problem which faces this country. The medical profession will have to accept this new expanded role on the part of this fellow group of health professionals; and I think that they will, to the ultimate benefit of us all.[30]

The conference addressed a number of important issues but really answered none. It was clear that, in spite of the talk, there was not a health care team nor were the roles and talents for the team even agreed upon by the various professions and practitioners. Pharmacy was challenged to address the lack of congruence between what the pharmacist was educated to do and what he did. More basic was the challenge to understand whether the pharmacist should be doing what he was doing—were some functions better left to a less-educated individual while the pharmacist moved into new responsibilities? Participants were challenged to prepare for change because many were satisfied with the status quo, with traditional perks and privileges, and would be slow to see the need to change unless they were led and role models for the future provided.

ASHP-AACP Invitational Workshop

In 1971 the American Society of Hospital Pharmacists (ASHP) and the American Association of Colleges of Pharmacy (AACP) assembled representatives of sixty colleges of pharmacy, representatives of the two host organizations, and others to exchange information on the current status of clinical pharmacy practice and education. The hopes of the conference organizers and participants were, in part, to begin to establish a consensus on how the concept of clinical pharmacy would infuse new vitality into the profession.

Clinical pharmacy was widely perceived as being synonymous with hospital pharmacy. The belief was that the primary place where students would come into contact with clinical training was in the hospitals, not in retail or ambulatory practice. However, many colleges of pharmacy were not situated in a medical center and did not have access to a university hospital for training students. The first part of the Invitational Workshop provided perspectives of how the various schools were developing relationships to be able to provide patient-centered experiential training. The dissimilarity between these programs and the common need to educate students to begin to do things differently provides an insight into the developmental process of the period.

The editorial accompanying the report of the workshop posed three important considerations about the education and practice of clinical pharmacy that needed to be addressed.

1. There is an immediate need for pharmacy to critically evaluate, via the scientific method, the effectiveness of its practitioners in new roles which are encompassed by "clinical pharmacy." . . . Testimonials which relate all of the wonderful things that pharmacists can do, but which offer no proof, are not enough.

2. "It is essential that we convince the public, other health practitioners, health planners, administrators, and legislators that the clinical component is essential but will increase the cost of pharmacy education significantly." ... Even more pressing, perhaps, is the need to convince the public and legislators of the value of comprehensive pharmaceutical services if reimbursement for such services as well as for drugs is to be included.

3. Restructuring pharmaceutical education is likely to have little future unless education of the pharmacist is integrated and coordinated with that of physicians, nurses, and other health professionals.[31]

Communicating the Value of Comprehensive Pharmaceutical Services to the Consumer

In 1972, the American Pharmaceutical Association commissioned the Dichter Institute for Motivational Research to learn more about the perceptions and beliefs of American consumers about pharmacists. The study was done with over 500 consumers in twenty-three states. Each consumer had to have had at least two prescriptions filled within the past four months. This study was undertaken in large part because of the changes in health care, including the provision of pharmaceutical products, and how those changes were affecting the pharmacist-patient relationship. The final report, *Communicating the Value of Comprehensive Pharmaceutical Services to the Consumer,* was published in 1973.

The key concept identified by the study was that the consumer felt alienated by the pharmacist. In the absence of a personal relationship with their pharmacist, any pharmacist would do. This insight explained why patients were leaving the community pharmacy in favor of the mass merchandisers and discount houses. In addition to the lack of contact, data showed the lack of communication between the pharmacist and consumers.

> We find that the pharmacist has lost contact with his patients. We find, too, that patients expect—and, indeed, want—contact, personal attention, and professional services from the pharmacist. ... The public is almost completely in the dark as to what the pharmacist really does. One of the public's most prevalent perceptions is that the pharmacist hides behind a specialized coun-

ter in a corner of the establishment, makes a little bit of noise
and comes up with a small bottle and a large bill. The public
must be told about the extreme care the pharmacist must take.
. . . We are not unaware of the theory that the pharmacist is
unique in that he can both be a tradesman and a professional.
Nowhere else in the patient's frame of reference is there a professional who doubles as a tradesman. And because the patient
has no frame of reference in which to adequately position and
understand the pharmacist's dual role as a tradesman and a professional, the theory is dysfunctional.[32]

This conclusion led the investigators to identify the establishment of
a strong level of communication between pharmacists and patients as
the single most important outcome of the study.

Manpower

In the 1949 Survey, the issue of manpower was placed in the very
first section of the recommendations. The country was just emerging
from a depression and the war. Enrollment in the colleges had been
restricted and an unknown number of pharmacists lost. There were no
complete data on the availability of pharmacists to know whether the
demand for pharmaceutical services could be met. Using the data
available from the National Association of Boards of Pharmacy and
the estimated need for new pharmacists and the capacity of the
schools to train them, Elliott projected a potential national shortage of
approximately 10,000 pharmacists. The report went further than establishing a quantitative need, however. The report also began to establish a qualitative measure as part of the manpower requirements.

Pharmaceutical operations at all stages are undergoing many
and considerable changes. The professional manpower must be
constantly ready to cope with these changes—educationally,
economically and ethically. . . . Briefly stated, the manpower
problem is the problem of putting the whole of the house of
pharmacy in such a condition as to be livable, economically and
professionally, for pharmacists prideful of their profession.[33]

Health care grew as a national policy issue. As the population expanded there was increasing need for health professional manpower

to also grow. In 1961, the federal government introduced the Health Professionals Education Assistance Act which provided assistance to medical and dental schools. In the mid-1960s, Medicaid and Medicare were passed and put into effect. The demand for health care that emerged quickly increased and, with it, the demand for more health care professionals. Senator Warren Magnuson and Congressman Paul Rogers were the champions of the effort to have pharmacy included in the Health Manpower Act of 1968. Their support was based on the belief that pharmacists had much to contribute to improved health care. They also were well aware of the development of clinical pharmacy initiatives in a number of the colleges.

What emerged from the Health Manpower Act of 1968 were capitation grants that were intended both to increase enrollment and to improve education. Funding was based in part on the increased head count over a previous base. The Special Projects Grants portion of the program were to assist schools

> in meeting the cost of special projects to plan, develop or establish new programs or modifications of existing programs of education in such health professions or to effect significant improvements in curriculums of any such schools or for research in the various fields related to education in such health professions, . . . or to assist any such schools to meet the costs of planning experimental design thereof, or which will otherwise strengthen, improve, or expand programs to train personnel in such health professions or help to increase the supply of adequately trained personnel in such health professions needed to meet the health needs of the Nation.[34]

Many schools utilized part of the capitation funding to begin or expand clinical pharmacy programs. However, there were still important issues that had to be addressed, such as where to find qualified teachers, what should the curriculum look like, and what will clinical pharmacy deliver to society. Brodie, then on a special assignment with the Department of Health, Education and Welfare, was a driving force in putting together the Invitational Conference on Pharmacy Manpower held in San Francisco in 1970. This program focused its attention not on the quantitative needs of expanding manpower, but rather on the "how and what" that the new pharmacist should be capable of doing.

Though still in its infancy and viewed more or less as a "laboratory curiosity," a clinical role for the pharmacist emerged as a subject of major interest. Information was shared about new concepts and programs being initiated in a number of schools of pharmacy. However, in the absence of a definition for this role beyond that of being a "patient-oriented one," the following imperatives evolved during the conference: First, develop working criteria to describe the role. Second, test its effectiveness. Third, determine if it is economically a feasible role or under what conditions it is feasible. For the first time, also, the Conference provided the pharmacy profession a comprehensive outline of current needs.[35]

There was little agreement or homogeneity in the approaches that schools took in developing their clinical pharmacy programs. Likewise, the needs and expectations of the constituency of the schools were different. Some saw clinical pharmacy as relevant only in the hospital setting and in a PharmD program. Others saw the concept of clinical pharmacy as a basic component of the move toward patient-oriented practice. Some schools were located in a university health center setting where interactions with other health professionals in a hospital setting were facilitated. Many pharmacy schools, however, were separated from other health professional schools or were the only health program within the university. The need for models to show how the challenge to prepare future practitioners might be met was essential. The 1971 American Society of Hospital Pharmacists and the American Association of Colleges of Pharmacy invitational workshop provided a forum for the sharing of different experiences in the development of programs and the establishment of criteria for faculties.[36] In 1972, the American Association of Colleges of Pharmacy sponsored a report that collected a state-of-the-art picture of clinical pharmacy education in four prototype pharmacy curricula (University of California–San Francisco, University of Minnesota, Purdue University, Washington State University). Criteria for these programs were

1. a setting in which pharmacy education is integrated with that of other health professionals in a university medical center complex;

2. a setting in which pharmacy and medical education coexist on a common campus;
3. a setting in which the pharmacy school is isolated from any of the health professions.[37]

The quantitative issues of manpower were still of concern, partially because of the need to gain a complete census of the profession but more importantly to answer the question of the Health Manpower Act. The American Association of Colleges of Pharmacy undertook an ambitious program to do a census of the profession and gain a snapshot of the tasks that practitioners were engaged in. As part of this project, AACP worked with the individual state boards of pharmacy to obtain a voluntary census of practitioners and their sites of practice. The second phase was to understand what pharmacists were really doing in their practice. An important conclusion was that pharmacists already in practice would need to increase their interactions with patients. This finding suggested that pharmacy education would have to expand educational efforts to practitioners as well as students if there was an expectation that clinical pharmacy would be widely available to impact patients' health care.[38]

Significance of the Conferences.

The twenty-five-plus year interim period between the publication of the Elliott Report and the Dichter Report was a busy one for pharmacy leadership. There were over a dozen various surveys, task forces, and invitational conferences that were devoted to questions relating to the pharmacist's role, education, and place in health care.

In this period there was also a marked change in the perspective and the focus of the inquiries. The period begins with a professional self-examination, the Elliott Report. In this effort, the focus was by pharmacy, on pharmacy, and for pharmacy. The core questions were what did pharmacists do and how should professionals be educated and regulated for those tasks. By the time of the Dichter Report, there was a 180 degree shift in perspective. Now it was the time for patients, the consumers of the pharmacist's services, to articulate what the pharmacist needed to do in order to meet the public's needs and expectations. The debate and dialogue of the interim years were critical in bringing this change about.

All of the issues that were identified and explored during the interim years can be generalized into three broad, but still interrelated, categories. These were (1) the isolation of the pharmacist, (2) product focus rather than patient focus, and (3) relevance of pharmacy in a time of change. Other issues such as degree title and curriculum content were widely debated, but they were not the core issues which had to be resolved before any meaningful changes for the profession of the future could be broadly implemented. The conferences went beyond merely cataloging issues. They identified and began to build agreement, if not consensus, on the concept with the potential to provide solutions. This concept was clinical pharmacy, an interim step which helped to define a future role for pharmacists and the training that would be necessary to achieve its practice.

Isolation of the Pharmacist

The pharmacist was isolated in his practice, isolated from other health professionals, isolated from colleagues, and, most important, isolated from patients. This way of working began in the education and training that the pharmacist received and was replicated in practice.

While there was a vast amount of discussion about the need for the health care team in the interim period, pharmacists were not prepared for working and contributing to the team. Many schools were not located in a health care center where faculty and students could freely interact and be exposed to the contribution of the other professions. Even in those schools that were located in a medical center complex, such interactions were rare. The curricula of the different professions were based on different models, as Brodie pointed out in the 1964 APhA-ASHP Commission. Pharmacy followed the physical sciences, notably chemistry, while the other health professions followed the applied sciences, that is, applied to patients. The experiential training of pharmacy was in the dispensing laboratory or in the dispensing area of a pharmacy. The experiential training for the other health professions was at the side of the patient.

The pharmacist was isolated in practice, both geographically and in terms of his patients. Pharmacy has always been proud of the fact that pharmacists are the most available of all of the professions. This positive factor also had a downside. Many pharmacists practiced in small towns and in small stores. This left little time to continue learning from each others' experience and fellowship. Continuing education, frequently impersonal, was the mechanism that was put forward to allow those who wanted to keep current with advances to do so.

The pharmacist's isolation from the customer was well documented during the interim period. This started when the pharmacist was not trained to interact with patients. Remember, pharmacy was the only profession that did not have a "clinical" requirement. In the 1970 conference, "Challenges to Pharmacy," there was wide recognition that the economics of practice were pushing the pharmacists behind counters and away from patients. Furthermore, until this trend was reversed, additional training in patient orientation might be for naught.

Product Focus versus Patient Focus

Pharmacy was the only health profession that was reimbursed for its sale of a product rather than for its provision of a service. The pharmacist practiced in a mercantile establishment, and one that was not even wholly dedicated to the sale of health items. The pharmacist was paid for the sale of a product, a product which may or not be a medicine. Finally, the pharmacist was moving from the direct view of the patient. Hidden behind a counter, the patient had no sense of what services the pharmacist might or should provide beyond selling a medicine that he couldn't get anywhere else. Frequently, the merchant portion of the profession was perceived as more important than the professional services, especially since it was more evident. This dilemma was identified in almost every study in the interim period, whether that study was solely for pharmacists, from an interdisciplinary perspective with other health care professionals, or with patients. Perhaps the Dichter Report summarizes it best by calling out the fact that this mixture of merchant and profession had no other model and therefore was dysfunctional.

Relevance of Pharmacy in a Time of Change

Health care was in a period of change and reexamination during the interim years. There was a growing realization that medicines were powerful agents that helped but also had the power to hurt. There was an awareness that many of the hospital admissions were due to adverse drug reactions, some of which could be avoided. Patients were becoming more vocal about taking an active part in their health care. One of the public's issues was access to the best health care that their insurance could buy. The maldistribution of physicians and other health care providers was a public policy issue. Finally, health care was an expensive proposition and the payers, especially the government, wanted to be sure that they were getting what they paid for.

During the period, pharmacists often described themselves as "overeducated and underutilized." The bachelor's degree had been expanded to a five-year program, but this did not bring much of a change to what pharmacists did. Instead of focusing on the patient and the biological and applied sciences, much of the time was still devoted to compounding and the basic sciences. This was in spite of the fact that compounding was a rapidly diminishing portion of the pharmacist's activities. The 1967 Pharmacy-Medicine-Nursing Conference noted that the needs of the specialist scientist were given priority over the professional goals of the students.

The question was raised, especially by Brodie, about the profession's willingness to make the hard decision and commit to change. This was not an easy observation but it was a critical one. If the profession could not, or would not, change and become recognized for its expertise by both other health care professions and the public, it would regress to a position of a technician.

Clinical Pharmacy

Clinical pharmacy, at its strongest, was a concept that was intended to answer the issues that had been identified in the intervening years and move pharmacy to a higher, more professional plane. The concept was to move pharmacy, in education as well as in practice, to a patient-centered profession. The AACP definition of clinical pharmacy recognized that the curricula must focus on patient care with an emphasis on drug therapy.

The period was a time of exploration and experimentation into what clinical pharmacy might be. From the first experiments at the University of California–San Francisco College of Pharmacy grew an increasing interest in moving the pharmacist to the patient's bedside in an inpatient setting. A number of schools developed new curricula that would seek to expose students to patients as part of the requirements for graduation. Many times this change was not easy, especially for schools outside of a medical center complex. These programs had to find and build relationships with hospitals and institutions where there may not have been a preexisting relationship. However, clinical pharmacy was a means, rather than the end, to achieve the professional shift that was needed. The underlying question was what would the clinical pharmacist do, what would be contributed to the health care team and society that otherwise would not happen.

That answer was provided by Brodie in the concept of "drug-use control." Brodie stated that the "ultimate goal of the service of pharmacy must be the safe use of drugs by the public."[39] This single statement was a powerful rationale for the clinical role of the pharmacist and the promise of what this individual would deliver and to whom it would be delivered. Drug-use control uniquely answers the challenges posed by the issues facing pharmacy. In order to practice clinical pharmacy, interdependency with the rest of the health care team is required. Isolation is impossible when the pharmacist has responsibility for a component of patient care. The patient is the basis for the product, rather than the reverse. The need to deliver the right medicine to the right patient is more than the responsibility of handing over the product. There is a need to see that the product is used to obtain the desired end.

The PharmD Debates

The length of the period of education and what the terminal degree should be called were not new debates in the period leading up to the Millis Commission. Indeed, in the twentieth century, pharmacy education had moved from an apprenticeship and a few weeks of part-time education to one year, to two years (PhG), to three years (PhC), to four years (BS). The Elliott Survey specifically recommended a six-year, doctor of pharmacy (PharD [sic]) program. However, that recommendation was not implemented and, in 1960, a compromise was reached for the five-year BS.

There were a number of issues in the PharmD debate. These included whether the degree should be an entry-level professional doctorate or an advanced, specialized degree; what the length of time of the educational program should be; and what skills would be required for the faculty of new courses. Also, there was the question of what these graduates would do and where they would practice.

Inherent in the development of clinical pharmacy programs was the belief that pharmacists should have a patient focus. What was being debated was an ideological conflict of two positions. The first was that clinical education, such as the Kentucky and Texas programs, was designed for specialized practice in hospitals and clinics while the other believed that the elements of clinical practice should be available to all patients. Adherents to the former position held that the PharmD was a graduate degree, received as a consequence of specialized, postbaccalaureate training. It was believed that the pharmacist would practice in an institutional setting as part of an interdisciplinary patient care team that included physicians. Proponents of the latter position held that the degree was an entry-level degree. They claimed that clinical education was a necessary component for the education of all pharmacists in order to provide a basic level of service to patients in any setting, no matter whether it be a small town, a metropolitan chain drug store, or a clinic or institution.

To be clear, there was not universal support for the PharmD degree regardless of whether it was the first degree or a graduate degree. There still was no consensus on what roles the pharmacists of the future would need to be prepared for nor how to train them for those roles. The faculties, largely composed of basic scientists, had to be convinced that clinical faculty were needed to develop new roles and that these faculty should have corresponding rank, privilege, and responsibilities. Practitioners were not convinced of the need for longer education nor what advantage it would deliver. The cry "overeducated and underutilized" showed the frustration that practicing pharmacists already had, and more education without a new role was not going to be the answer that alumni were interested in. Employers of pharmacists were also very resistant to the six-year PharmD. The expansion of education signaled a potential limiting of the labor pool, which would result in increased labor costs. Without a new role, and increased revenue stream from new skills, employers could see very little value in a new degree.

The focus of the debate rightly needed to be on the most important questions of what a pharmacist should do and what the curriculum should be to meet that goal. The debates during the intervening years reached the consensus that pharmacists, if they are to be fully integrated health professionals, must focus on the patient and must be prepared to deliver a service that exceeds simply providing a product. Once the patient focus role was articulated and understood, it was time to move forward with developing the curriculum that would enable the faculties to prepare students for the role. The question of what to call the degree is probably the least important part of the debate.

Changes in the practice of pharmacy are, in large measure, reflections of the education pharmacists receive during their college education. Ideas for changes in practice are not necessarily conceived within the colleges, but the evolution and status of change is dependent on the educational program. The concept of educating pharmacy students for a role that included patients and other health professionals was developed and expanded during the 1960s and 1970s within the colleges.

THE CHARGE

Origins of the Millis Commission

The development of clinical pharmacy at the University of California–San Francisco, the University of Kentucky, and other leading educational programs and its rapid spread within the curricula of U.S. colleges of pharmacy during the 1970s was stimulated by a perceived need to make the practice of pharmacy an essential part of the changing health delivery system. Health care leaders, from pharmacy as well as other professions, believed that pharmacists could and should be important contributors to the improvement of both the quality and availability of health care. However, these changes were threatening to many pharmacists who worried about how changes envisioned would affect their place and security with the profession. Perhaps because the introduction of clinical pharmacy was often identified as both the savior and culprit in the controversy, because clinical pharmacy had its origin within the colleges, and because there was a division within faculty members as to the place clinical pharmacy should have in practice, AACP became the natural leader of efforts to initiate a study to better understand and communicate the future role of pharmacists.

During its interim meeting in 1969, Alan Brands, then the pharmacy liaison officer to the U.S. Public Health Service, challenged the AACP Board during his review of the Task Force on Prescription Drug Report. While his comments were largely devoted to the question of manpower availability, he also spoke of the Task Force recommendation: "Pharmacy education has a responsibility of preparing not only for the present but also for the future, even innovating for the future and guiding the course of the profession."[40] The board picked up this recommendation and moved to establish a "subcommittee of the Executive Committee to prepare a grant application for review by the Committee for funds with which to undertake a study of pharmaceutical education."[41]

Reports from the subcommittee were given to the executive committee at each of the next five meetings during the period of 1969 to 1971. Proposals for the project were revised and studied, but support for them was not secured. Clearly, another course of action needed to be developed if a study was to become a reality. This action was set into motion by A. E. Schwarting in his presidential address to the AACP annual meeting in 1972. At that time he put forward the resolution to establish a Commission on Pharmacy, composed of health providers and consumers, to make a study of pharmacy and pharmacy education to determine the scope of pharmacy services in health care and the necessary education process:

> The time is *now* for an in-depth study and evaluation on pharmacy and pharmacy education. This study should 1) identify the needs of society for appropriate drug therapy and related pharmaceutical services and acknowledge the deficiencies in health care as they relate to these services, 2) identify role models to fulfill these needs in concert with the functions of other health professionals, 3) define the nature and structure of future programs to educate these practitioners, and 4) define the manner by which these findings should be disseminated.[42]

The Study Commission on Pharmacy

In October 1972, The American Association of Colleges of Pharmacy invited John S. Millis to form a commission and serve as its chair. In September 1973, with full funding secured, the Study Commission met for the first time. The final session of the Commission was in September 1975 and the full report, *Pharmacists for the Future,* was published in December of that year. The Study Commission was quickly identified with the chair as "the Millis Commission."

POSTSCRIPT

It was impossible to review the period between the completion of the Elliott Survey and the Study Commission on Pharmacy and ignore the contributions of Donald C. Brodie. His presence, contributions, and leadership to the profession were both many and significant. Dr. Brodie dedicated his life to the delivery of health care with emphasis on the roles of the pharmacist. His most important platforms were in the areas of pharmacy education and practice. He was constantly challenging those of us who are health care professionals to join efforts that would save precious dollars and increase the quality of health care for the patient. He constantly stimulated, some say challenged, us to address our recognized weaknesses in order to better serve society. Dr. Brodie's candor and belief took the high ground that the profession had to "do good" by meeting its societal mission in order to "do well" for itself.

> America at mid-twentieth century finds two of its great institutions—medical care on the one hand, and education on the other—in the throes of dramatic revolution. At work in each are numerous small revolutions—revolutions of ideas, of technology, of practice, of attitudes, and of goals. Underlying these enormous eruptions are two clearly distinct but inter-related entities—people and knowledge. Great numbers of people are to be served; vast and ever-increasing stores of knowledge are to be interpreted and used. So vast and complex has become man's accumulated knowledge, that few comprehend the magnitude and significance of it all.[43]

NOTES

1. E.C. Elliott, *The General Report of the Pharmaceutical Survey, 1946-49* (American Council on Education, Washington, DC, 1950), p. 3.

2. E.C. Elliott, *The General Report of the Pharmaceutical Survey, 1946-49* (American Council on Education, Washington, DC, 1950), p. 98.

3. E.C. Elliott, *The General Report of the Pharmaceutical Survey, 1946-49* (American Council on Education, Washington, DC, 1950), pp. 229-230.

4. E.C. Elliott, *The General Report of the Pharmaceutical Survey, 1946-49* (American Council on Education, Washington, DC, 1950), p. 218.

5. "The Seminar Number," *Am. J. Pharm. Educ., 14:* 5-6, 77-157 (1950).

6. L.E. Blauch and G.L. Webster, *The Pharmaceutical Curriculum* (American Council on Education, Washington, DC, 1953), p. 246.

7. L.E. Blauch and G.L. Webster, *The Pharmaceutical Curriculum* (American Council on Education, Washington, DC, 1953), p. 247.

8. D.C. Brodie, *The Challenge to Pharmacy in Times of Change* (The American Pharmaceutical Association and the American Society of Hospital Pharmacists, Washington, DC, 1966), p. 1.

9. D.C. Brodie, *The Challenge to Pharmacy in Times of Change* (The American Pharmaceutical Association and the American Society of Hospital Pharmacists, Washington, DC, 1966), p. 39.

10. D.C. Brodie, *The Challenge to Pharmacy in Times of Change* (The American Pharmaceutical Association and the American Society of Hospital Pharmacists, Washington, DC, 1966), p. 39.

11. D.C. Brodie, *The Challenge to Pharmacy in Times of Change* (The American Pharmaceutical Association and the American Society of Hospital Pharmacists, Washington, DC, 1966), pp. 42-43.

12. D.C. Brodie, *The Challenge to Pharmacy in Times of Change* (The American Pharmaceutical Association and the American Society of Hospital Pharmacists, Washington, DC, 1966), p. 44.

13. D.C. Brodie, *The Challenge to Pharmacy in Times of Change* (The American Pharmaceutical Association and the American Society of Hospital Pharmacists, Washington, DC, 1966), p. 45.

14. D.C. Brodie, *The Challenge to Pharmacy in Times of Change* (The American Pharmaceutical Association and the American Society of Hospital Pharmacists, Washington, DC, 1966), p. 48.

15. D.C. Brodie, *The Challenge to Pharmacy in Times of Change* (The American Pharmaceutical Association and the American Society of Hospital Pharmacists, Washington, DC, 1966), p. 49.

16. D.C. Brodie, *The Challenge to Pharmacy in Times of Change* (The American Pharmaceutical Association and the American Society of Hospital Pharmacists, Washington, DC, 1966), pp. 4-5.

17. R.A. Deno, *Proceedings of the Pharmacy-Medicine-Nursing Conference on Health Education* (University of Michigan, Ann Arbor, MI, February 16-18, 1967), pp. 28-29.

18. R.A. Deno, *Proceedings of the Pharmacy-Medicine-Nursing Conference on Health Education* (University of Michigan, Ann Arbor, MI, February 16-18, 1967), p. 35.

19. R.A. Deno, *Proceedings of the Pharmacy-Medicine-Nursing Conference on Health Education* (University of Michigan, Ann Arbor, MI, February 16-18, 1967), p. 81.

20. R.A. Deno, *Proceedings of the Pharmacy-Medicine-Nursing Conference on Health Education* (University of Michigan, Ann Arbor, MI, February 16-18, 1967), pp. 92-93.

21. H.F. DeBoest, *Proceedings of the Third Professional Pharmacy Seminar* (The Lilly Research Laboratories, Indianapolis, IN, 1969), p. 16.

22. H.F. DeBoest, *Proceedings of the Third Professional Pharmacy Seminar* (The Lilly Research Laboratories, Indianapolis, IN, 1969), p. 140.

23. H.F. DeBoest, *Proceedings of the Third Professional Pharmacy Seminar* (The Lilly Research Laboratories, Indianapolis, IN, 1969), p. 166.

24. H.F. DeBoest, *Proceedings of the Third Professional Pharmacy Seminar* (The Lilly Research Laboratories, Indianapolis, IN, 1969), p. 171.

25. H.F. DeBoest, *Proceedings of the Third Professional Pharmacy Seminar* (The Lilly Research Laboratories, Indianapolis, IN, 1969), p. 175.

26. D.C. Brodie, *Challenge to Pharmacy in the 70s: Proceedings of an Invitational Conference on Pharmacy Manpower* (University of California, U.S. Department of Health, Education and Welfare, Washington, DC, 1970), p. v.

27. D.C. Brodie, *Challenge to Pharmacy in the 70s: Proceedings of an Invitational Conference on Pharmacy Manpower* (University of California, U.S. Department of Health, Education and Welfare, Washington, DC, 1970), p. 113.

28. D.C. Brodie, *Challenge to Pharmacy in the 70s: Proceedings of an Invitational Conference on Pharmacy Manpower* (University of California, U.S. Department of Health, Education and Welfare, Washington, DC, 1970), p. 7.

29. D.C. Brodie, *Challenge to Pharmacy in the 70s: Proceedings of an Invitational Conference on Pharmacy Manpower* (University of California, U.S. Department of Health, Education and Welfare, Washington, DC, 1970), pp. 77-78.

30. D.C. Brodie, *Challenge to Pharmacy in the 70s: Proceedings of an Invitational Conference on Pharmacy Manpower* (University of California, U.S. Department of Health, Education and Welfare, Washington, DC, 1970), p. 55

31. "Proceedings of the ASHP-AACP Invitational Workshop on Clinical Pharmaceutical Practice and Education" *Am. J. Hosp. Pharm., 28:* 841-906 (1971).

32. Dichter Institute for Motivational Research, Inc., *Communicating the Value of Comprehensive Pharmaceutical Services to the Consumer* (American Pharmaceutical Association, Washington, DC, 1973), pp. 14-15.

33. E.C. Elliott, *The General Report of the Pharmaceutical Survey, 1946-49* (American Council on Education, Washington, DC, 1950), pp. 211-212.

34. G.L. Webster, "Address of the President," *Am. J. Pharm. Educ., 32:* 377 (1968).

35. D.C. Brodie, *Challenge to Pharmacy in the 70s: Proceedings of an Invitational Conference on Pharmacy Manpower* (University of California, U.S. Department of Health, Education and Welfare, Washington, DC, 1970), pp. v-vi.

36. "Proceedings of the ASHP-AACP Invitational Workshop on Clinical Pharmaceutical Practice and Education" *Am. J. Hosp. Pharm., 28:* 841-906 (1971).

37. *Clinical Pharmacy Education and Training Program: A Special Report* (American Association of Colleges of Pharmacy, Washington, DC, February 1972).

38. *Pharmacy Manpower Information Project* (American Association of Colleges of Pharmacy, Washington, DC, 2 vols., 1972).

39. D.C. Brodie, *Challenge to Pharmacy in the 70s: Proceedings of an Invitational Conference on Pharmacy Manpower* (University of California, U.S. Department of Health, Education and Welfare, Washington, DC, 1970), p. 39.

40. "Minutes of the Interim Meeting" *Am. J. Pharm. Educ., 33:* 298 (1969).

41. "Minutes of the Interim Meeting" *Am. J. Pharm. Educ., 33:* 299 (1969).

42. A.E. Schwarting, "Address of the President: Some Propositions for Progress," *Am. J. Pharm. Educ., 36:* 351-355 (1972).

43. D.C. Brodie, *The Challenge to Pharmacy in Times of Change* (The American Pharmaceutical Association and the American Society of Hospital Pharmacists, Washington, DC, 1966), p. v.

Chapter 3

New Insights into the Commission

Dennis B. Worthen

The title for the final report of the Study Commission on Pharmacy, *Pharmacists for the Future,* reflects both the work and the workings of the Commission over the two years that it was in existence. The title was chosen late in the very last meeting of the Commission. The discussion recalled that this was a citizens' commission that would report its findings not only to pharmacy educators and the profession but also to the entire health care system, including its users. The title selected for the report said it all. It communicated the need to look forward rather than backward and broadly signaled that this work was not just for pharmacists but rather for all interested in health care delivery. Once suggested, the title was immediately accepted by the individual Commission members. The common insights gained during the two years that the Commission met helped the members develop a shared vision of two things: what a profession could contribute to societal good and the belief that their report could help achieve that goal.

The eleven meetings of the Commission were a group learning process that focused on exploring what was happening in pharmacy and what was planned or foreseen for the future. This learning approach brought to the surface the aspirations and vision of leaders and practitioners as well as the perspective of how the profession of pharmacy saw itself fitting into the health care delivery system. The Commission also met with others involved in delivering health care, including physicians, nurses, regulators, and manufacturers. These individuals provided a perspective of how they saw pharmacy's role in the health care system and how well pharmacy was delivering relative to societal needs. This group learning process, which was developed by Millis, was effective. It developed the articulation of what the future for pharmacists might be; the reality check to see if it was right from the perspective of the profession's health care partners; and the conclusions of what needed to be done to deliver the promise of the vision.

BEGINNINGS

The Study Commission is a visible marker of the change in the profession. Earlier studies, such as the milestone Charters and Elliott reports, focused on pharmacists and what they did, or needed to do, as pharmacists. They were internally oriented, designed for pharmacists, and did not seek or accommodate the needs or requirements of the society served. The studies did address the questions of how pharmacists can do better that which pharmacists do when they do pharmacy. For the most part the profession was not studied from a societal perspective that asked the questions of what should pharmacists do. By the late 1960s, pharmacy had matured to the point where the internal issues were well in hand and the perspective started to change to the broader societal role of the profession.

The shift to a societal perspective can be glimpsed in a number of places in the years leading up to the Study Commission. Several examples of this are the Pharmacy-Medicine-Nursing Conference on Health Education at the University of Michigan in February 1967 and the consumer study by the Dichter Institute for Motivational Research that the American Pharmaceutical Association commissioned. In his American Association of Colleges of Pharmacy (AACP) presidential address, Schwarting made the case for pharmacy education to formalize this new perspective of pharmacy as a part of the health care system and to develop an understanding of the role of pharmacists within that system and what they would need to know in order to be successful.[1]

An AACP committee chaired by Schwarting developed a white paper that provided the basis for the new study. The first element was the increasing need to address the misuse of drugs—both licit and illicit. Drug abuse of substances such as amphetamines and heroin was increasing. Drug misuse due to poor compliance or incomplete understanding of the proper use of medicines was resulting in hospital admissions or longer hospital stays. The second element was the call from some outside of pharmacy to study whether the pharmacist, trained as a drug specialist, could or would be a more useful member of the health care team. Both abuse and misuse were identified as major contributors to the rapidly increasing cost of health care. More important, the need or opportunity for pharmacy to fill a new role was evident. The AACP white paper served as the briefing document in discussions with potential chairs and became part of the charge to the Study Commission itself.[2]

Does education lead practice or does practice lead education? This professional version of which comes first, the chicken or the egg, was in evidence both in the AACP committee and later in the Study Commission. While there were clear signals that society had new needs that providers of health care, including pharmacy, needed to meet, there was no clear or overwhelming response to those signals. The challenge to develop a vision of what society needed and how pharmacy might position itself to fill that need fell to education. In order to meet that challenge, the Study Commission on Pharmacy addressed itself to developing a vision for the future, not a mirror to the past.

THE STARTING POINT

In a memorandum to the Study Commission members which served as a starting point for the first meeting in September 1973, Millis laid down the general priorities that the Commission needed to address. He then shared what he termed the "Anomalies of Pharmacy." These anomalies followed his definition of pharmacy only to conclude that, while the broad definition of pharmacy may be the "invention, development, manufacture, distribution, prescription, and dispensing of biological and clinical agents used in the cure, control or prevention of disease,"[3] the meaning of pharmacy conveyed to most people is much narrower.

The first anomaly was specialization. Most health care professions became more specialized as a result of expanding scientific and technological advances. The fields of medicine and surgery developed along lines of gender, age, body part, and disease. Dentistry moved from a "drill and fill" orientation to prevention and divided itself into specialty areas such as orthodontia and periodontia. Dentists were involved in all of the specialties. Nursing likewise moved into specialty areas such as anesthesia and surgery. Again, nurses were involved in all of these specialties. Pharmacy, on the other hand, developed along the lines of research and development, manufacture, distribution, and dispensing. However, unlike the other health professions, pharmacists were not involved in all of the special areas; only dispensing remained as the professional function.

The second anomaly was a consequence of the new scientific and technological knowledge that placed limitations on who could do what. Physicians are licensed to do almost anything that physicians do. That is, once physicians are licensed they can do any diagnosis, therapy, and surgery. Their activities are not limited by their license but rather by the restrictions imposed by the institutions where they practiced, their own knowledge of their capabilities, and potential sanctions and malpractice threats. Thus, in spite of the flow of new knowledge about potent new pharmaceutical agents, there were no restrictions placed on the use of them. Any licensed practitioner could use any medicine available on the market.

Social and political forces were similar for pharmacy and medicine in most instances. The major difference emerged in the economic domain where physicians, dentists, and nurses are paid for delivering a needed and valued service. The value is the skill which is difficult to measure and impossible for anyone else to deliver. The pharmacist, on the other hand, delivers a product. While this process may also require a skill, it is easier to identify the product and presume that almost anyone can meet the requirements for delivery.

PHARMACY: THE PERSPECTIVES

There is some evidence that Millis began his work for the Commission by trying to identify the most important questions, including where to begin and where to focus deliberations. One of the most important questions was whether the investigation was concerned with pharmacy, including the pharmacist, or with the pharmacist. Millis goes on to state:

   a. I can see no choice. To start with a preconceived definition of
      the pharmacist would lead only to a selection of bits and pieces
      which in turn would create gaps and lead to obsolescence.

b. It would be better to see the universe of pharmacy and define (insofar as we can) the pharmaceutical roles of all kinds of professionals. Then see what kind of functions cannot be so assigned and define the pharmacist from this.[4]

This question, perhaps, best articulates the strategy of perspective: whether the beginning point for the Commission should be pharmacists looking out at what they could and should do or society looking in at what could and should be done. While subtle, this strategy is important, and one of the hallmarks of the Millis Commission.

If the Commission had begun its deliberations based on the pharmacist's perspective, what might have emerged? It is possible, even probable, that the Commission would have focused on items of self-interest to the profession, including use of technicians, third class of drugs, and the entry-level degree. Instead, by focusing on the societal perspective, the Commission developed a broader definition of pharmacy, identified the patient as the justification for existing, and described knowledge rather than product as the basic professional deliverable.

While somewhat redundant, it is important to paint a historical perspective of the profession in the early 1970s. From the pharmacist's perspective, the measure of how well he performed was whether or not the right patient got the right product at the right time. It was inappropriate, if not illegal, for the pharmacist to discuss the therapy with the patient; instead, the patient should be directed back to the physician to get information and answers. The public perceived pharmacists more as businessmen who "hide behind a specialized counter in the corner of the establishment" than as a health care professional.[5]

The Commission developed the perspective that the basic definition of pharmacy needed to be expanded to incorporate the concept of communication of knowledge within the health care system and that the system includes the patient. While the traditional definition of pharmacy as a compounding and dispensing profession was accurate, it was limiting. Practice had changed markedly over time, and especially in the post–World War II era. Pharmacists no longer compounded many prescriptions; that function had become the provenance of the manufacturer. The need to prove the safety and efficacy of the product was also the domain of the manufacturer. The pharmacist's domain had largely become the distribution of the product, the interim step between the manufacturer and the patient. However, pharmacy was a health service that could be considered a knowledge system—just like medicine, dentistry, and nursing. To accomplish the move to this perspective, pharmacists would need to broaden their focus from only product distribution to include disseminating knowledge and information about the product in order to achieve a desired outcome. That outcome was the dissemination of information on medicines within the health care system so that knowledge and products "contribute to the health of individuals and the welfare of society."[6]

DELIBERATIONS

There were eleven meetings of the Commission between September 1973 and September 1975. In that period there were over 6,000 pages of transcription of the group's deliberations; in addition, there were numerous papers, statements, and exhibits by the various consultants who were meeting with the Commission. At the conclusion of each session, Millis prepared a set of précis which captured the essence of the discussion and provided the basis for the final report. The engaging question is what were the pivotal points or insights that influenced the Commission in the group learning exercise that had been set for it? While that question is difficult to answer with certainty, the following are likely:

- The pharmacy system is different from the rest of health care.
- The nature of pharmacy is dichotomous.
- Current education is not sufficient to deliver required step changes.
- Therapy is changing from treatment to prevention.
- It's the patient.

Pharmacy Was Different from the Rest of Health Care

Of course it was! The important differences were not between the obvious factors of dispensing versus prescribing; they were with the basic orientation of the profession. Therein lies the question of what the basic mission, and education for that mission, needed to be.

Perhaps the biggest, or most obvious, difference between pharmacy and the rest of health care in the period leading up to the Study Commission was pharmacy's orientation to product rather than patient. This orientation was being challenged by the spread of the concept of clinical pharmacy. The best known example of this was the twelfth-floor unit at the University of California–San Francisco, where the education of pharmacists was being incorporated with other health professionals at the patient's bedside. Course work was predominately devoted to chemistry, pharmacology, and even pharmacognosy. Every hard science had multiple laboratories. Curriculum changes resulting from the Elliott Survey focused largely on compounding and dispensing, in spite of the fact that compounding was rarely practiced anymore. Even the compromise addition of a fifth year of education did little to move the pharmacist away from compounding and product. While some liberal arts courses were added to the curriculum, they were largely restricted to the first two years of preprofessional education. Communications skills were not integrated with basic sciences to build a model of how to communicate with other health care professionals or patients.

While there may have been professional connections between the faculty of the pharmacy school and its sister units in the health care center, only about a third of the pharmacy schools were part of an academic health care campus. There was no mingling of students of the various professions to learn a model for the delivery of health care in a system.

> Pharmacy education has been an education in isolation. Even those of us in academic centers who are students rarely go outside the walls of the building we are in, never interact, for example, with patients, never interact with other health professionals, never interact in a structured way with our own professional men out in practice.[7]

Pharmacy education did not include patients. The laboratories and course work focused on the product. What the product was made of, how it was made, and how it worked was the core focus of education. Every other health profession—medicine, nursing, and dentistry—focused on the patient both to deliver their skills and then to see how their art and science affected the patient. An essential part of professional education was time on the wards and in clinics to learn how to interact with, and care for, the patient to a particular outcome.

This orientation was due, at least in part, to the direction that emerged from the two earlier hallmark studies, Charters and Elliott. The focus was noted by Jere Goyan in his presentation to the Study Commission during the first meeting. He reviewed the early works and noted that they attempted to bring pharmaceutical education up to the standards of their time. However, they were driven by the needs of the profession, not by the needs of the individual patient or society. It was clearly a time for shifting the orientation of the profession, but the question remained where to shift. Goyan finished his remarks with the following:

> When we first asked Jack Millis to assume the Chairmanship, he asked, "Has pharmacy reached a stage of divine discontent which would enable the report of such a Commission to have a positive impact on the future of your profession?" We answered with an unqualified "yes."[8]

The Dichotomous Nature of Pharmacy

The dichotomous nature of pharmacy was a critical dilemma: Was pharmacy a mercantile business or a professional service? There was the need to separate the perception, if not the reality, of the pharmacist as the businessman from the pharmacist as the professional, while still providing enough income to make the professional role economically viable. In addition, society needed to have better health care, including more involvement from pharmacists, without increasing overall costs.

The questions of what a pharmacist was and what he did were central for Millis from his earliest discussions with the AACP committee. Likewise, they were recurring questions for the full Commission. At issue was whether the pharmacist was a professional dealing with patients and within the health care system or a businessman caught up in the need to make a profit on the products he sold. The confounding factor was that not everything he sold pertained to health care. Products sold in the pharmacy included cosmetics, greeting cards, and other sundry merchandise found in hardware and other retail establishments. This question was not the unique province of the Commission; the question was also coming from some in the profession, from other health care professions, and from payers.

The Study Commission was aware of the Dichter Report. This study had been commissioned by the American Pharmaceutical Association and had the stated purpose of determining how to communicate the value of comprehensive pharmaceutical services and to increase demand for the services from the public. Two basic questions were explored in an attempt to meet this objective: Does the consumer know that these services are available, and are they of value? The field research took place in 1972 and the final report was issued in 1973.

The key findings must have been disturbing. Data indicated that the pharmacist had lost contact with his patients and, as a consequence of this loss, price rather than professional service became the criterion to choose the place to get prescriptions filled. The concept of "push/pull" was put forward. Patients felt "pushed" away by their feelings of loss and alienation from their community pharmacist. In turn the patient was "pulled" to the lower-price provider because there was no difference in the satisfaction for the services obtained.

Finally, the theme that came up frequently in the discussions of the Commission was the schizophrenic positioning of the pharmacist between professional and merchant. The question really came down to whether someone could sell general merchandise one moment and deal with serious health issues the next. The question also dealt with the ability to provide professional services in a site that looked like a "big top tent."

> The pharmacist has lost his professional standing primarily because the patient cannot visualize him as a tradesman and a professional simultaneously. Even the type of establishment in which pharmacies are usually located detracts from the pharmacist's professionalism, since physicians and lawyers and dentists perform their services in offices.[9]

Current Education Is Not Sufficient to Deliver Required Step Changes

The education of pharmacists was the central theme for the Study Commission. All of the efforts of the Commission focused on discovering what the profession should be doing, not on what it had been doing. This is not to imply no attention was paid to the past. Even if the Commission wanted to focus on the future, many of the consultants who spoke to the Commission focused on the past and defended what they were doing. The consultants' vision of the future was frequently very short term and was stated in terms of the past rather than in aspirations for the future.

The Commission was faced with several challenges, including the need to determine where the health care needs of society would be in the future. The parallel challenge required an understanding of the differentiated strengths of the profession and how these might be developed to meet the identified societal needs. Differentiated strengths are those that can be uniquely provided by practitioners because of education, training, and knowledge. They are not strengths that are recognized solely through a regulatory monopoly. The regulatory monopoly can be changed with varying degrees of ease while knowledge must be acquired.

Brodie and Weston

Two consultants to the Commission, Donald C. Brodie and Jean K. Weston, perhaps best articulated the potential and the need for changes in the educational process for pharmacy. These two individuals were the only consultants to meet privately with the Commission, and for an extended period of time. Each was an expert in his field. However, their perspectives of the role and value of what was then called the "clinical pharmacist" were diametrically opposed. In that opposition, these two men represented both the emerging search for a new professional mission and the push of the health care team, as represented by the physician, to limit that expansion.

Donald Brodie was a pharmacy educator. At the time of the Study Commission, Brodie was working with the Department of Health, Education and Welfare in Washington. He had taught for a number of years at the University of California–San Francisco and had been a major force in the establishment of the clinical floor at the University Hospital. Brodie has been widely credited with the development of the concept of "drug use control." This concept is defined as "the sum total of knowledge, understanding, judgments, procedures, skills, controls, and ethics that assures optimal safety in the distribution and use of medication."[10]

Jean Weston was a researcher and physician. He taught neuro-anatomy before joining the pharmaceutical industry as a researcher. Later, he joined the American Medical Association in the Division of Drugs and worked on the first edition of *AMA Drug Evaluations*. When he was giving a presentation at the School of Library and Information Science at Case Western Reserve University, Weston met Millis and discovered a common interest in drug information.

Don Brodie met with the Commission during the second session in November 1973. During the session, six pharmacists, each working in a different practice site, talked about their practices. The pharmacists were asked to respond to three questions:

1. What does the pharmacist do?
2. What could the pharmacist do that he does not now do?
3. What should the pharmacist do?[11]

The six practitioners held views that were strongly influenced by the environment they worked in. As they identified the challenges of their practice, however, communications with physicians emerged as a consistent issue; even those pharmacists who practiced in the same institution as the physician identified this as an issue. Community practitioners also identified patient compliance as a particular concern, and this certainly represents a communication problem between the professional and the patient. Brodie then summarized his general impressions of the comments of the six:

> We did not see a very clear or concise portrayal of the moving frontier of pharmacy thought and action. . . . It came through clearly as to what they are doing now. I had hoped to see a little more imagination. There is now one basic question which no one has ever asked. What are the deficiencies and economics or lack thereof in the existing drug distribution and use process?[12]

In his private time with the Commission, Brodie suggested that pharmacy must be viewed in the broader context of the health care delivery system. He based this position on three assumptions that provide the rationale for considering the pharmacist as part of the system. The first assumption was that the drug component of health care is a subsystem of the entire health care system. The second was that the drug component is an essential component of health care. The final assumption was that the drug component was composed of two functions—distribution and service. He argued that each provider in the health care system is responsible for part of the process and that pharmacists were responsible for the drug component. However, there were issues, such as those identified by the practitioners in the earlier session, that made the pharmacist less effective than he should be.

Brodie was concerned about the isolation of pharmacists during their education. The lack of common training leads to poor communications and lack of understanding of what each provider can contribute to the overall good of the health care system.

> Health professionals must be trained together if they are going to work together effectively. I see in my past no coming together of the health professionals. I am convinced that we have to see to it that the students in the health disciplines must have overlapping degrees and education.[13]

The message was clear and forceful. If pharmacy did not integrate within the health care system, it would be difficult for the decision makers in the system to consider pharmacy as a partner, and pharmacy would be the worse for the isolation. This was a challenge for education where less than half of the schools were in a medical center environment and a greater challenge in practice as noted by the six practitioners who identified communications—both with physicians and patients—as a common issue. Brodie pointed out that the communication skills of the pharmacist must be improved and a common terminology developed. For the pharmacist that meant a vocabulary that was more consistent with heath care terminology than drugstore terminology.

Brodie concluded by identifying the issues that he thought were the most critical for pharmacy:

1. How does the concept of pluralism in the care delivery system apply to pharmacy and pharmacy education?
2. There is a need to direct the focus of pharmacy on the needs of the patients for drug related services and away from the focus on the place where the service is rendered. "We need to get the pharmacists out of the drugstore and into the practice of his profession."
3. The need to improve the accountability of the pharmacist.

4. The need to avoid a dual system of pharmacy education—to bring the concepts of distribution and service together.
5. The need to improve the pharmacist's capacity in communication. This requires the development of a vocabulary which is health service oriented.
6. The need to be concerned with the efficiencies and economies of pharmacy.
7. The patient, the least qualified person, is making the most important decisions about drug therapy. Patient compliance is therefore a central problem.[14]

Jean Weston met with the Commission during the seventh session in November 1974. Unlike Brodie, Weston did not sit in on the presentations of physicians. Instead, his meeting followed two half-day meetings with the leadership of professional and trade pharmacy associations. Consequently, his comments did not build off of testimony that he heard with the Commission members.

Weston described the physician as the individual responsible for patient care, which is composed of two facets—diagnosis and therapy. Further, these two components are inextricably linked in an iterative process. That is, without continuing diagnosis and feedback, therapy is not optimized. He posed one question, in three different ways, that challenged a basic tenet of the clinical pharmacy movement which professed responsibility for a patient's therapy. One version of the question was:

> Put still a third way, how would the pharmacist's education and experience be further modified to permit him to play what additional part effectively in the actual care of patients, now that pharmacy professes to be clinically oriented and to deal with patients rather than customers.[15]

This question raises three points that were critical issues to the ability of pharmacy to move into the future: (1) what education is required; (2) what is effective patient care; and (3) can pharmacy really move from a commercial, customer orientation to a patient focus?

Weston began by reviewing the education that medical students received compared to the clinical pharmacy students. First, the number of hours that medical students spent in patient-related activities was enormous. From at least the last two years of medical school through the experiential training in the internship and residency, patients were the focus of the medical student. Beyond the number of hours, however, was the question of the teachers involved.

> Reviewing the clinical qualifications and experience of the "clinicians" who teach medical students as compared to those who teach clinical pharmacy students readily makes clear the far superior clinical qualifications of the medical school teachers in most instances, excepting in those relatively few where the same clinicians teach both type of students. The relatively recent survey of the clinical pharmacy curriculum by Pitlick and Plein, both academic pharmacists, makes apparent how woefully little time is spent in "clinical" pursuits by even the few schools classed by the authors as superior in this regard. It further verifies that the "clinical" qualifications of their teachers can not compare with the "clinical" qualifications of medical school teachers therapeutically or probably in any other way.[16]

Weston goes on to point out that the quality of the individuals in clinical pharmacy was good. There was no question of their intelligence, dedication, or ability. What was missing was sufficient clinical experience to qualify the pharmacist to take responsibility for the patient's therapeutic management.

The issue of effective patient care is one that reverts to serving the patient's best interests. The role of the pharmacist should be as a team member, under the physician's supervision and control. Several roles were suggested that the pharmacist would be well qualified to fill. One was the provision of drug education. This role would be to develop drug information services that would be available to all health care professionals to facilitate appropriate use of therapies. Furthermore, the same, or a similar service, should be provided to patients to help them maximize their therapies. Another role would be in specialized areas of therapy such as that developed by Robert Maronde with hypertensive patients in ambulatory care at the University of Southern California.

During his prepared remarks, Weston did not return to the question of whether pharmacy could really move from a customer orientation to a patient focus. However, the question was reflected in the entire discussion relative to what should the pharmacist do in the future that is generally not being done today. Is the patient the mission of pharmacy or is product distribution and provision its mission?

Leighton Cluff, a physician member of the Commission, later returned to the question of trying to define clinical pharmacy. He posed the question, "to what purpose, where, how, and by whom is training in clinical pharmacy conceived," and then answered it as follows:

Purpose	To prepare the pharmacist to provide that knowledge and information about drugs in an effective and appropriate way to the patients and prescribers, pertinent to the settings where patient care is being provided.
To what degree	To the degree that will provide the pharmacist sufficient familiarity with patients and their problems to allow him to dispense a drug and appropriate information about the drug to the patient.
How	Clinical training can be provided only by participation in the health care process.
By whom	At the present time by physicians, nurses, and behavioral scientists since at the present time there are no appropriately experienced pharmacists to do so.
Where	Those settings in which pharmacists can experience and contribute to the care of patients—namely, in clinical settings where other health professionals are learning about patients and where health care is being provided.[17]

Brodie and Weston arrived at the same conclusion. In spite of the fact that Brodie was a major proponent of the clinical pharmacy movement and Weston was a proponent for continuing physician control, their conclusions were strikingly similar. In order for pharmacy to move to being truly patient focused, pharmacists must have the right education. This education must be provided by faculty qualified to teach their areas of expertise. However, there were few faculty who could fill the shortage of clinicians in pharmacy education. The role "requires the discipline of vigorous research at the point of delivery of pharmacy services and a thorough knowledge of one or more of the basic pharmaceutical sciences."[18] Most important, pharmacy must become interdisciplinary in education if it is ever to become interprofessional in practice. A new practice model for all of the health professions is the patient-centered health care team. If pharmacists are not trained as part of the team, it will be very difficult for them to act as part of the team when they enter practice.

Therapy Is Changing from Treatment to Prevention

Pharmacists identified themselves, and were identified by others, with the products that they were responsible for, but these products were changing. These changes carried new opportunities and challenges for society and for pharmacy. In effect, the therapeutic armamentarium was moving from its focus on the treatment of disease to one that was focused on maintaining health. During the ninth meeting in March 1975, Bryce Douglas put the idea of "social drugs" forward to the Commission as a significant force that could alter pharmacy and pharmacists.[19]

Douglas was not referring to drugs of abuse, or substance abuse, when he talked about social drugs. Instead, he was identifying products that focused on prevention and early detection of disease. He was also referring to an area that included health issues rather than illness issues. Specific examples that he suggested included the entire area of contraception, products that were used to avoid pregnancy rather than terminate it. He also included products that could be used to facilitate intellectual facility, including tranquilizers and stimulants. Finally, he identified those agents that might be used to deal with substance abuse, whether that abuse be other drugs, alcohol, or tobacco.

Jan Koch-Weser suggested that the term "social drugs" was inappropriate but that the concept was accurate. These drugs are taken by healthy people to achieve a personal end, such as pregnancy avoidance or increased mental activity. As such, this was an area where

> the pharmacist could play a very central role and very important role because here the information about the drug is all-important; the information about the person who takes the drug is much less important because we are dealing with healthy people. . . . the fact that he [the pharmacist] does not know as much

as the physician does about tumors of the ovary is really beside the point because the physician has already determined that this particular patient does not have a breast cancer or a tumor of the ovary.[20]

There were other changes noted in therapeutics area. While significant progress had been made in curing communicable disease, less progress had been made with degenerative conditions—those conditions frequently associated with aging, hypertension, diabetes, cardiovascular disease, and cancers. Research, both in industry and academia, was being focused into the areas of chronic diseases. Douglas noted that cardiovascular diseases were receiving 70.1 percent of the research and development budget in industry.[21] His conclusion was that the future health care system would have to be capable of dispensing not only the products, but the knowledge for the proper use and understanding of them, to assure proper use and patient benefit.

The two trends, that of social drugs and that of focusing on the treatment of degenerative conditions, were joined in the concept of quality of life of the patient.

> . . . one of which is the quality of life—whatever that means. I believe you used the word "health." Fundamentally, that is an acceptable term with you but you are really talking about the concern as to the quality of living rather than the necessary mortality per se. Perhaps it is the realization that until we do understand the aging process, and presently I don't think we understand it at all, there is going to be increasing emphasis upon concern of the quality of living rather than mortality.[22]

It's the Patient

From the beginning, Millis asked a series of questions that would guide the Commission in its deliberations. In a memorandum that he sent to the Commission members before the first meeting, he noted that the Commission must answer four questions:

a. Who should be educated?
b. How many should be educated?
c. How should they be educated?
d. For what should they be educated?[23]

He went on to add that the final question, for what should they be educated, was the most important one. The answer that emerged from the very beginning was clear and unmistakable: pharmacists must be educated for the patient.

The first meeting of the Commission was important for setting the stage for the study. Some of the members met one another for the first time. The entire first day of the meeting was devoted to learning why they were called together and what this task was they had agreed to take on. AACP staff and committee provided an in-depth survey of what had transpired in earlier studies—not just the Charters and Elliott studies—but all of the past self-examinations. The second day was devoted to deciding how the task would be approached. Millis summarized the first day as the prelude to the task:

> Yesterday it was said and I think, it was generally accepted, that the great need is to look at pharmacy from the point of view of the patient—that is, unless we come up with something which deals with people, not pharmacists, not research laboratories, not physicians, not nurses, not drug store proprietors, not the system, et cetera, we really have not added much. . . . I would like to see the patient and improvement of health by utilization of drugs be the focal point of our considerations and also not forgetting all of the other participants in the chain because, obviously when we talk about what he does do now, what could he do, and how do you train him to do that, we are not talking just about the relationship of the pharmacist to the patient but we are talking about the pharmacist's relation to the nurse, the relationship of the pharmacist to the physician, the relationship of the pharmacist to the manufacturer, the relationship of the pharmacist to the distributor and then, to a certain extent, there is another element in the whole system and that is governmental regulation.[24]

The role of the chairman is to set a course and lead. That is precisely what happened here. It is not that others would not have considered the patient as the focal point of the study but the direction was clearly set. The answer to the question of what the pharmacist should be educated for was "for the patient."

During several sessions, consultants addressed issues surrounding patients. One of the recurring themes was the lack of the patient's compliance with the therapeutic plan established by the physician. Interestingly, the picture of the patient that comes through from the discussion was more of an object that could be ordered to follow instructions than a participant in the delivery of health care. This suggests that if there was one group that the Commission should have heard from, and didn't, it was from patients themselves. John Biles highlighted the omission of patients in a summary of the pharmacy practitioner meeting.

> We also heard that the patient determines whether or not his prescriptions should be filled by the pharmacist. In the example of polypharmacy we heard that the patient determines what fraction number of his prescriptions written should be filled and that the fractional number filled is determined on the basis of cost. We heard that prescriptions filled by the pharmacists were not picked up by the patients. The least qualified individual is therefore making decisions regarding drug therapy. It occurred to me during the presentations by the visitors that teamwork, the provision of pharmaceutical care, and the utilization of the pharmacist's knowledge of drugs in the clinical environment was more advanced in the institution than in the community or professional pharmacy.[25]

The word *patient* historically referred to someone who was ill and under a professional's care. This definition no longer works in an environment where health is the focus rather than illness. In the discussion about "social drugs," Bryce Douglas made the point that these new therapies were not just to take care of sick people but to obtain some other, personal end, such as contraception and memory enhancement. This trend requires that pharmacists become even more willing and able to provide information to people who medicate to their own ends, and even self-medicate through the use of nonprescription medicines and alternative medicines.

Who is the pharmacist working for—the customer or the patient? While never explicitly stated, this question appears to be one of the underlying complexities that the Study Commission had to work through. Certainly, there was a great deal of discussion around the pharmacist's role as a storekeeper and small businessman. Within that role the proper term was likely to have been customer, because the pharmacist is selling a product. The orientation more clearly shifts to patient when the pharmacist is providing a service that adds value to the health care system. A clear case can be made when, for example, the pharmacist is providing information about products that will help the patient use the product appropriately and avoid unnecessary problems.

Finally, the vision for pharmacy had to change. Health care itself was changing and pharmacy needed to be better integrated with the broader system. The old way of doing things didn't deliver all of the value possible to the patient. Too often the phrase "overeducated and underutilized" was being applied to the profession by its own practitioners. The broader health care system was asking what pharmacists really added, other than serving as intermediaries for product distribution. Simply providing a product, even if it was a potent and valuable medicine, was not an acceptable role for the pharmacist as a health care professional in the changing world. There was a need to move the profession from being product centered to one that was patient centered. The problem with many therapies was not that the product didn't work; it was that the patient didn't use it appropriately to gain the desired outcomes. Focus of the health care system, including pharmacy, had to move to where the problem could be addressed and corrected—and that is the patient.

THE COMMISSION

In 1973, twelve individuals came together to form the Study Commission on Pharmacy. The Commission members were from diverse backgrounds. There were pharmacists, physicians, educators, and a nurse. They worked in academia, in industry, and in practice. In retrospection, the common bond between the individuals was that they were all well educated and each was involved in health care in some way. They were, to fit Millis's requirement, individuals given to thinking, learning, and understanding. Sitting as a committee-of-the-whole, they heard from a large number of individuals who shared their perspectives of what pharmacy was, or wasn't; what it should or should not do; and how to educate students to perform their role at an appropriate level of competence.

The groups and individuals who presented to the Commission represented virtually every special interest group within pharmacy. This included practitioners, educators, regulators, and practicing pharmacists. In addition, physicians and nurses spoke on their experiences with pharmacists. External forces to pharmacy, such as representatives of the Food and Drug Administration, the pharmaceutical industry, and representatives of institutions, such as hospitals, provided perspectives of the profession and its practitioners. In the end, over eighty individuals met with the Commission.

The Commission also had access to information on the history and progress of the profession and literature not only from pharmacy but from all of the health professions. All of this was to assure that the Commission would have as much information about the profession and the challenges that it faced as possible.

The task that awaited the Commission was not simply to summarize and organize the input of the consultants and then provide it to the sponsor and funding organizations. Rather, the task was to develop a sense of what society needed to have the pharmacist do in the future and how the pharmacist should be educated to meet that challenge. The very process of the Commission interacting within itself was a strong exercise in developing learning and understanding. Since the Commission was a learning organization, it was to be expected that they would produce a new sense of what was possible rather than validating what was already accomplished.

> But, as one who was there, I was equally or more impressed by the contributions of most of my Commission colleagues. The Commission members were there to listen and learn and discuss and seek consensus on the identification of important issues and the formulation of recommendations, but they spent as much or more time discussing and learning from each other than they did with the 80 odd consultants and the guts of the Commission report came from the Commission not the consultants. I am convinced that I learned much more from my Commission colleagues than from the relative[ly] brief exposure to the consultants.[26]

SUMMARY

Pharmacists were an isolated group. They were not educated with the other health professions; they did not have clinical experiences with patients; and they practiced, for the most part, in relative isolation. They were not integrated in the larger health care system and consequently were frequently treated as outsiders. Many complained that they were poorly treated by the system and that the system didn't value their contributions, but pharmacy was not perceived as a contributing part of the system. Pharmacy was perceived by its practitioners and users alike as a distribution system for products rather than as a profession that had the capability to work within the system to deliver a unique benefit to the ultimate user, the patient.

In the position paper "A Case for a Study of Pharmacy Practice and Pharmacy Education," the AACP committee laid out the case for the need to change.[27] Health care was having problems with medications. There were too many admissions to hospitals due to misadventures; hospital stays were too long because of misadventures; and the costs attributable to these misadventures were too high, too predictable, and preventable. There was clearly a societal need for something to be done to address this problem. The clear question was who, which health care profession, would take on the challenge. It was clearly a time when society could no longer accept the status quo in terms of how medicines were used in the health care system.

This was the challenge that the AACP committee articulated, but the need for change was also felt within the profession itself. Victor Morgenroth articulated that need at the end of the session with pharmacy practitioners. While speaking for himself, he summarized the practitioners' testimony to the Commission:

> we were hung up with tradition and I think if we can do one thing within the Commission it is, for heaven's sake to get rid of that first and start from here because if we do not and we do not stop thinking about what happened then we will never make progress. . . . today we find the whole system being changed and if we don't change with it as a profession, then we shall, in turn, cease to exist.[28]

Perhaps it was this sense of societal and professional consequences that focused the Commission on the future rather than on past. The past was done and could not be undone, but the future could be shaped by the lessons and knowledge gained from the past. The consultants to the Commission provided a clear picture, from their individual perspectives and vested interest positions, of the gaps within the health care system that offered opportunities for pharmacists to engage with the system. Perhaps this opportunity can best be stated by noting the axiom that states that in order to achieve a "breakthrough" one must first "break with."

NOTES

1. A.E. Schwarting, "Address of the President: Some Propositions for Progress," *Am. J. Pharm. Educ., 36,* 351-355 (1972).

2. *Drug Misuse: The Pharmacist and the Physician* (later retitled: *A Case for A Study of Pharmacy Practice and Pharmacy Education*), University Archives, Case Western Reserve University, Classification # 1DD9, Box 41.

3. J.S. Millis, "Memorandum to Members of the Study Commission on Pharmacy," August 13, 1973, University Archives, Case Western Reserve University, Classification # 1DD9, Box 42.

4. J.S. Millis, undated, handwritten note, 4 pp., University Archives, Case Western Reserve University, Classification # 1DD9, Box 43, Folder 1.

5. Dichter Institute for Motivational Research, Inc., *Communicating the Value of Comprehensive Pharmaceutical Services to the Consumer* (American Pharmaceutical Association, Washington, DC, 1973), p. 14.

6. *Pharmacists for the Future: The Report of the Study Commission on Pharmacy* (Health Administration Press, Ann Arbor, MI, 1975), p. 14 [p. 156].*

7. W. Kinnard, Transcript of First Meeting, September 13-14, 1973, University Archives, Case Western Reserve University, Classification # 1DD9, Box 46, Folder 1, pp. 112-113.

8. J.E. Goyan, Transcript of First Meeting, September 13-14, 1973, University Archives, Case Western Reserve University, Classification # 1DD9, Box 46, Folder 1, pp. 40-52.

9. Dichter Institute for Motivational Services, *Communicating the Value of Comprehensive Pharmaceutical Services to the Consumer* (American Pharmaceutical Association, Washington, DC, 1973), p. 41.

10. D.C. Brodie, *The Challenge to Pharmacy in Times of Change* (The American Pharmaceutical Association and the American Society of Hospital Pharmacists, Washington, DC, 1966), p. 39.

11. Notes from the Second Meeting, November 16-17, 1973, American Association of Colleges of Pharmacy Papers in the American Institute of History of Pharmacy Collection at the State Historical Society of Wisconsin, Madison, WI, Mss # 293, Box 167, Folder 6.

12. Notes from the Second Meeting, November 16-17, 1973, American Association of Colleges of Pharmacy Papers in the American Institute of History of Pharmacy Collection at the State Historical Society of Wisconsin, Madison, WI, Mss # 293, Box 167, Folder 6, p. 23.

13. Notes from the Second Meeting, November 16-17, 1973, American Association of Colleges of Pharmacy Papers in the American Institute of History of Phar-

*Bracketed pagination refers to pages in Appendix A.

macy Collection at the State Historical Society of Wisconsin, Madison, WI, Mss # 293, Box 167, Folder 6, p. 20.

14. Précis II-2, Second Meeting, November 16-17, 1973, University Archives, Case Western Reserve University, Classification # 1DD9, Box 43.

15. J.K. Weston, *The Relative Therapeutic Training and Likely Real Therapeutic Competence of Physicians and Para-Physician, Especially the Pharmacist, in Modern Patient Therapy,* American Association of Colleges of Pharmacy Papers in the American Institute of History of Pharmacy Collection at the State Historical Society of Wisconsin, Madison, WI, Mss # 293, Box 167, Folder 11.

16. J.K. Weston, *The Relative Therapeutic Training and Likely Real Therapeutic Competence of Physicians and Para-Physician, Especially the Pharmacist, in Modern Patient Therapy,* American Association of Colleges of Pharmacy Papers in the American Institute of History of Pharmacy Collection at the State Historical Society of Wisconsin, Madison, WI, Mss # 293, Box 167, Folder 11, p. 3.

17. Précis IX-3, Ninth Meeting, March 7-8, 1975, University Archives, Case Western Reserve University, Classification # 1DD9, Box 45.

18. Précis IX-3, Ninth Meeting, March 7-8, 1975, University Archives, Case Western Reserve University, Classification # 1DD9, Box 45.

19. Précis IX-2 and Transcript, Ninth Meeting, March 7-8, 1975, University Archives, Case Western Reserve University, Classification # 1DD9, Box 45 and Box 49, pp. 339-383.

20. Transcript of Ninth Meeting, March 7-8, 1975, University Archives, Case Western Reserve University, Classification # 1DD9, Box 49, pp. 675-676.

21. Transcript of Ninth Meeting, March 7-8, 1975, University Archives, Case Western Reserve University, Classification # 1DD9, Box 49, p. 352.

22. Transcript of Ninth Meeting, March 7-8, 1975, University Archives, Case Western Reserve University, Classification # 1DD9, Box 49, p. 356.

23. J.S. Millis, "Memorandum to Members of the Study Commission on Pharmacy," August 13, 1973, University Archives, Case Western Reserve University, Classification # 1DD9, Box 42.

24. Transcript of First Meeting, September 13-14, 1973, University Archives, Case Western Reserve University, Classification # 1DD9, Box 46, pp. 304-305, 314.

25. J. Biles, "Comments Regarding the Proceedings of the Meeting of 11/16/73," given on November 17, 1973, University Archives, Case Western Reserve University, Classification # 1DD9, Box 43, Folder 2.

26. R. Straus, Personal Communication to D.B. Worthen, September 4, 1997.

27. "A Case for A Study of Pharmacy Practice and Pharmacy Education," University Archives, Case Western Reserve University, Classification # 1DD9, Box 41, Folder 6.

28. Transcript of Second Meeting, November 16-17, 1973, University Archives, Case Western Reserve University, Classification # 1DD9, Box 46, p. 386.

Chapter 4

Reactions to the Study

Marie A. Abate

BACKGROUND

The Millis Study Commission on Pharmacy attempted to answer the question of what the appropriate education for pharmacists in the future, including the 1990s and the year 2000, should be. It examined the health care system, the relationship of pharmacy to this system, and provided a number of recommendations for the practice and education of pharmacists. Although the content of the report was not completely new or innovative, many of the predictions in the Millis Commission report later came into being and many of the ideas proposed were subsequently implemented. In fact, several of these predictions have been occurring gradually over time and many of the recommendations are still in various stages of implementation. After reading the Millis report and reflecting on the present practice of pharmacy, one can only conclude that change is often very slow in occurring.

The Study Commission's predictions, ideas, and recommendations were broad in scope and involved among other topics the role of the health service delivery system and changes in this system, the focus of pharmacy practice and education, the future direction of pharmacy services, and drug information provision. They concluded that pharmacy was ineffective and inefficient in developing, organizing, and distributing knowledge and information about drugs. Indeed, they felt that the greatest deficiency of pharmacy was in its inadequacy as an information transmitting system to physicians, other health care professionals, and patients.[1]

The focus of this chapter is on the early years following the Millis Commission's report, from 1976 until early 1981. Before examining the reactions by pharmacy education and practice during these first five years, however, it is useful to look at a few of the report's findings and relate them to occurrences in the present day.

THE PRESENT

The Millis Commission indicated that the health service delivery system of the future will become an information as well as a service provider. According to the report, the requirements needed for this change to occur included more effective communication between health professionals and patients, more effective communication between health care professionals of all types, utilization of new information systems and sophisticated information handling technology, and alteration in the education of health professionals so they learn to transmit appropriate knowledge and information.[2] These requirements appear to be met, at least partially, among the current health care professions. The Millis Commission also indicated that hospitals

> will probably expand their outpatient services; they will add ambulatory clinics. Large group practices may initiate HMOs. ... Health maintenance organizations will continue to appear in many alternative forms. The proportion of health services furnished by such organizations will continue to increase.[3]

These predictions have also come true in recent years; the development of HMOs and the services provided continue to expand throughout the country. The Millis Commission also stated that there will be increased future emphasis on both primary care and preventive medicine;[4] in fact, the health professions have only recently focused on these areas.

Other futuristic predictions of the Millis Commission pertaining to pharmacy practice included a requirement for pharmacists to monitor patient and institutional drug utilization,[5] an increasing use of pharmacy technicians,[6] the payment of pharmacists for total drug services whether or not they include dispensing,[5] and the use of computers, sophisticated technology, and effective communication systems for drug information provision.[7] Again, each of these predictions now represent important components of contemporary pharmacy practice.

In the education area, the Millis Commission predicted that the future pharmacy curriculum might necessitate awarding a degree higher than the baccalaureate degree.[8] The present move by schools and colleges of pharmacy to an entry-level doctor of pharmacy degree is evidence of this prediction's validity, although recommendations to develop a six-year curriculum had actually come forth two decades earlier than the Commission's report.[9,10] The Commission also felt that the best method to use for designing a new curriculum is one based upon desired competencies in the graduates,[11] and that the skills of problem identification, problem solving, and continued learning were essential to such a curriculum.[12] In his commentary about the report, Harold Wolf agreed that academia needed to identify appropriate competencies for graduates as an initial step in pharmacy curriculum development. Although work in this area had begun, Wolf stated that "much remains to be done to resolve this primary issue." Furthermore, although mentioned in the report, he felt that insignificant emphasis was given to the importance of incorporating active student learning and self-study throughout the curriculum.[13] The importance of producing pharmacy students who are critical thinkers, problem solvers, and motivated self-learners is now widely recognized in pharmacy education.

Finally, although the term "pharmaceutical care," in which the focus of pharmacy services is on the patient, is a relatively new one, the concept is not. When speaking of the clinical pharmacy movement at that time, the Study Commission indicated that the emphasis of clinical pharmacy was on drugs and their utilization by the patient. They felt that attention must be paid to both the drugs and the patients for future pharmacists, in contrast to a focus primarily upon the drug product.[14] Thus, the Study Commission advocated pharmaceutical care provision not only in the institutional setting, the focus of the newly emerging clinical pharmacy profession, but in all areas of pharmacy practice.

THE EARLY YEARS

During the years 1976 through the beginning of 1981, evidence of both the turmoil affecting the pharmacy profession and the relevancy and potential impact of the Millis Study Commission on Pharmacy's report became apparent. Numerous articles in the literature attempted to predict the future of pharmacy practice,[15,16,17,18] identified the challenges facing pharmacy in the future,[19,20,21,22] and spoke of the changes in pharmaceutical education necessary to prepare pharmacists for future practice.[10,23,24,25] It is also clear from some of the literature of this time that pharmacy was not a unified profession with regard to its leadership,[9,20,23] nor was it widely respected by the public.[16] Patients were said to be unaware of the qualifications and expertise of pharmacists and were not obtaining the information that they desired.[26] Furthermore, studies found patient drug monitoring and counseling by pharmacists to be inadequate.[27] Many of the topics addressed in the pharmacy literature during the early years following the Study Commission's report reflected the same issues and concerns that the report itself addressed, providing at least indirect evidence that the report was widely read and its findings considered seriously.

THE YEAR 1976

Several articles published during 1976 addressed the future of pharmacy practice and the ideas proposed in the Millis report, although not all felt that the report was valuable. Donald Francke felt "that the Millis Report failed to explore the issues facing pharmacy to the depth that they require before any meaningful change can take place."[27] In contrast, Wolf believed that the report raised "hard issues" that would influence the pharmacy profession, even though specific details for a change process were not provided.[13] Similarly, William Kinnard referred to the report as a guide for the future.[23] He stated that pharmacy must decide those aspects of the report they agree with and implement them. An editorial published in early 1976 by George Archambault endorsed almost all of the report and indicated that it "may well be the turning point in American pharmacy."[28] His single disagreement with the Millis Commission's recommendations related to the training of pharmacy technicians. The Commission's report recommended that supervision of the education and training of pharmacy technicians should be the responsibility of colleges of pharmacy.[6] In contrast, Archambault felt that pharmacy technicians have been, and could be, trained successfully by more informal on-the-job programs.[28]

Archambault indicated that the burden for implementing the changes recommended in the Study Commission's report would be on the state boards and the schools and colleges of pharmacy; unless they took action, pharmacy practice would be condemned to one that was product, not patient, oriented.[28] Other publications in 1976 echoed the need for change in pharmacy education. Schools were told that they must work with pharmacy practitioners and provide assistance where needed, particularly with regard to the offering of continuing education programs based upon desired professional competencies and the development of a reimbursement system for pharmacy services.[23] It was also stated that the educational process must prepare students for a lifetime of change by emphasizing the need to become lifelong self-learners.[18,19] Another recommendation of the Study Commission that pertained to the educational system involved the need to train "clinical scientists" with the ability to apply scientific knowledge to the development of practice skills needed for providing patient services.[29] Kinnard, however, was not convinced of the need to create a clinical scientist, since he was unsure of the exact responsibilities of an individual of this type.[23]

Other publications during 1976 provided a number of recommendations and insights that paralleled those found in the Commission's report. Raymond Gosselin indicated that the interaction of the pharmacist and the patient would be the focal point for the provision of clinical pharmacy services.[18] H. N. Lunan similarly stated that the profession of pharmacy was moving in the direction of providing clinical, patient-oriented services.[19] Donald McLeod reviewed the literature regarding various clinical pharmacy functions, including those involving the drug use process, specific activities such as adverse reaction and drug interaction detection, management of the patient with hypertension, etc., as well as the development of clinical practice specialty areas, primarily in institutional settings.[30] Although many citations documenting these functions were provided, it was concluded that significant work remains before clinical activities become the standard for pharmacy practice in organized health care settings.

Interestingly, in his review of the literature McLeod did not mention the likelihood of clinical activities becoming the norm for community pharmacy practice.[30] However, Gosselin predicted that the greatest changes in the pharmacy profession would occur in the noninstitutionalized setting, involving ambulatory patients.[18] This view is consistent with the Millis Commission's prediction that out-patient services would expand in the future.[3] Kinnard believed that patient counseling must become part of routine pharmacy practice,[23] a feeling similarly expressed in the Commission's call for more effective communication between health professionals and patients.[2] Lunan further stated that in order for clinical practice to occur in community settings, enhanced communication skills for pharmacists were crucial.[19]

The Study Commission believed that the health service delivery system of the future would provide not only services but also information.[2] To accomplish this, they felt that more effective communication among health professionals was required, and this would necessitate new types of interdisciplinary cooperation and collaboration. Gosselin, in his article, stated that the physicians and pharmacists of the future would recognize the importance of providing each other with feedback regarding the drug therapy of individual patients. He felt that pharmacists and physicians need to develop a formalized system by which drug utilization reviews and assessments for individual physicians' practices could be performed.[18]

In his article, Kinnard raised the issue of the need for professional pharmacy organizations to work together to achieve the necessary changes in practice and education.[23] A lack of unity within and among these organizations was also cited by the literature in later years as being a hindrance to the profession.[9,10,22]

THE YEARS 1977 AND 1978

In 1977, Brodie addressed members of a Rho Chi chapter in which he referred to the Study Commission's report while focusing upon four specific issues: drug information services, professional judgment, the dual degrees in pharmacy education, and advocacy for pharmacy education.[10] With regard to drug information, he stated that "I hope that faculties in our schools of pharmacy grasp the full impact of what the Commission had to say regarding drug information." Students should learn how to use sources of drug information, the storage and retrieval systems for information, and how to communicate information to enhance patient care. Professional and clinical judgment must be used by pharmacists to apply their knowledge to individual patient care situations.[10]

In order to provide pharmacy graduates with the skills and knowledge necessary for patient-oriented practice, the Study Commission indicated that a degree higher than the BS degree might be needed.[8] In his address, Brodie agreed with this sentiment and felt that pharmaceutical education had been in a stalemate since 1950 when a six-year entry-level academic program was first rejected, and had been drifting in a primarily lateral (as opposed to forward) motion.[10] He further described a lack of advocacy for pharmacy education, with neither professional organizations nor the pharmacy profession as a whole serving as strong educational advocates. The stagnation of pharmacy was blamed on a resistance to change. Others echoed Brodie's belief that pharmacy lacked a powerful cohesive organizational structure.[9,22] David Krigstein, in his 1977 Remington Medalist address, felt that the absence of strong pharmacy leadership was the reason the profession did not achieve its full potential in the 1950s and 1960s and why it failed to adopt the recommendation to move to a six-year program.[9] Philip Sacks, outgoing APhA president at the time, also felt there was a lack of unity among pharmacy's leadership and called for pharmacy's "chaotic" organizational structure to be "revamped and revitalized."[22] It was concluded that long-term planning was needed by the pharmacy profession, and that enduring short-term hardships might be necessary in order to obtain future practice changes.

With the advent of drug product selection laws in several states, pharmacists needed to be accountable to the public. Early surveys being conducted were finding that pharmacists were not using appropriately their drug product selection authority.[22] During 1978, it was also apparent that the pharmacy profession had significant room for improvement with regard to the attitudes of its practitioners and the types of services provided. In a survey of Kansas pharmacists, half still felt that drug distribution represented the most important personal contribution of the pharmacist, while 48 percent considered drug information provision to be the most important contribution of pharmacists.[31] In a national survey of 815 hospitals, only 23 percent provided at least one of four identified clinical services.[32] Of the specific clinical services included in the survey, only 4 percent of hospitals obtained medication histories, about 11 percent performed patient counseling, 15 percent monitored the drug therapy of patients, and approximately 6 percent participated in medical rounds. Furthermore, only about 7 percent of the hospitals operated complete unit dose and IV admixture programs, had twenty-four-hour service, and provided at least one clinical service. It was concluded that, although advancement was shown compared to a prior survey undertaken in 1975, much improvement in hospital pharmacy practice was needed.

It was also during the years 1977 to 1979 that tangible evidence of the impact of the Study Commission's report appeared. In the Joint Commission on Accreditation of Hospitals' (JCAH) 1977 Standards for Pharmaceutical Services, clinical practice concepts were integrated throughout the document for the first time.[33] This is important in that the "Standards for Pharmaceutical Services" existed to provide a standard of practice for pharmacy. JCAH had drafted the revised updated standards and asked the American Society of Hospital Pharmacists (ASHP) for comment during 1976. The 1977 Standards were particularly significant in that the provision of drug information and other pharmacy services were included in addition to drug distribution and storage functions, which were the focus of past Standards. This shift in focus was consistent with the Study Commission's belief that future pharmacists must move away from emphasizing the drug product itself. The 1977 Standards also required pharmacist participation in in-service education and stated that the pharmaceutical service should provide patient instruction or instruction to nurses who advise patients about the correct use of medications. Although qualified by the phrase "within the limits of available resources," the Standards indicated that the pharmaceutical service should maintain a medication profile for each patient and review the patient's drug regimen for interactions or incompatibilities. Also for the first time, the Standards referred to the establishment of a drug information center within the health care facility.

Beginning in 1977, APhA issued yearly "Policy Statements on the Role of Community Pharmacy" that reflected those recommendations found in the Millis Commission report.[15] According to the 1977 Policy Statement, the practice of pharmacy should be defined as a patient-oriented service. The 1978 Policy Statement indicated that pharmacists have an obligation to contribute to patient education and should provide drug information to patients by a variety of methods best suited to the individual's needs. According to the 1979 Policy Statement, drug regimen review should be used by all pharmacists in all drug-therapy-related settings and adequate compensation should be provided to the pharmacists for this service. The 1980 Policy Statement indicated that clinical pharmacy services should be a part of health care programs developed and/or funded by agencies and organizations, and these services should be reimbursable. Furthermore, new Standards of Practice for the Profession of Pharmacy were developed from the 1978 APhA/AACP effort, "A National Study of the Practice of Pharmacy."[34] These standards of practice were officially endorsed by APhA in 1979 in another of its policy statements on the "Role of Community Practice," in which APhA also called for voluntary implementation of the standards into professional practices. The standards of practice addressed many of the recommendations made in the Millis Commission report and represented the basic responsibilities of pharmacists which were stated as "provide the cornerstone for the future practice of pharmacy."[34] The responsibilities in the standards of practice were divided into four sections. In particular, Sections III ("Patient Care Functions—Clarifies patient's understanding of dosage; integrates drug-related with patient-related information; advises patient of potential drug-related conditions; refers patient to other health care resources; monitors and evaluates therapeutic response of patient; reviews and/or seeks additional drug-related information")[34] and IV ("Education of Health Care Professionals and Patients—Organizes, maintains, and provides drug information to other health care professionals; organizes and/or participates in 'in-pharmacy' education programs for other pharmacists; makes recommendations regarding drug therapy to physician or patient; develops and maintains system for drug distribution and quality control")[34] reflected several of the activities called for in the Millis Commission report.

Other articles published in 1978 also reflected the thinking found in the Millis Commission's report.[21,35] It was stated by Herb Carlin, recipient of the 1977 Harvey A. K. Whitney Lecture Award, that comprehensive pharmaceutical services should be continuous, not episodic.[35] The motivation of pharmacists must be to service the needs of the patients, and pharmacists must be accountable for the services provided. When providing patient care services, Carlin believed that a patient-centered multidisciplinary approach, in which each health professional contributes to patient care as part of a team, was essential. This position was voiced in the Commission's report, in which it was stated that interdisciplinary collaboration and cooperative decisions among pharmacists and other health professionals were needed.[3]

Sister Duffy, in an address as then president-elect and vice chairman of the board of ASHP, expressed the need for hospital pharmacists to continue to develop and emphasize patient-oriented pharmacy services, particularly in smaller hospitals.[21] This was appropriate since clinical pharmacy services existed mostly in teaching hospitals during the 1970s.[36] Duffy stated that "we must make pharmaceutical services *relevant* to the health care program of the patient." She further indicated that the hospital pharmacy should make alterations in its practice to accommodate patient needs. In this regard, involvement in home health care was mentioned as a consideration.[21]

As mentioned previously, the Millis Commission in its report brought forth a concept that is well-recognized today as being important, that of competency-based instruction.[11] They felt it was best to begin to design a curriculum by clearly identifying and defining those functions that the pharmacist must do well, and then to develop the pharmacy curriculum in accordance with those competencies. In her paper, Sister Duffy agreed with the development of a competency-based curriculum and further stated that this concept should be applied to the development of continuing education programs.[21] She also specifically referred to the Commission's report when stating that hospital pharmacists need direction in order to progress, and to find this direction, they must determine the drug information needs of individuals and how to best provide the needed information.

The Study Commission referred to preventive medicine as being of increasing importance in the future and stated that it is both more effective and less expensive to prevent illness than to treat it.[4] However, they did not refer to the existing efforts of the pharmacy profession in the area of prevention. One 1978 commentary stated that pharmacy was clearly providing preventive health services, but that it must also evaluate and promote these services.[37] Examples of some of the preventive health services provided by pharmacists in the hospital environment included the development of the unit dose system to prevent medication errors, the use of centralized IV admixture services to decrease the infection risk, drug interaction monitoring programs, and efforts to increase patient compliance. However, the examples listed did not include such activities as pharmacist-provided patient coun-seling related to wellness and lifestyle changes and pharmacist-conducted disease state monitoring clinics.

THE YEARS 1979 TO 1981

Several publications during the years of 1979 to 1981 reflected a degree of frustration and discontent with the pace at which progress was occurring within the pharmacy profession. William Apple stated that pharmacy's spirit was very low, due to a variety of concerns.[20] These concerns included low salaries, a lack of opportunity for phar-macists to practice at their maximum abilities, a lack of recognition by the public, and less ability than in the past to become self-em-ployed. He felt that pharmacists often abandoned patients and failed to communicate with them. This led to patients who had no apprecia-tion of pharmacists' true knowledge and the role they could play in health care. Joseph Oddis in 1979 indicated that clinical pharmacy was still a concept of the future, due to a lack of acceptance in smaller hospitals and community pharmacies.[16] It was stated that although clinical and patient-oriented pharmacy services continued to expand at that time, there were still smaller hospitals and clinics and many community pharmacies which had yet to implement them. Phar-macists had become more involved in sales and merchandising and neglected the art of providing their drug knowledge to the patient. This led to a negative image of pharmacists in the eyes of the public. As an illustration, Oddis referred to wire service news stories that named pharmacists, along with garage mechanics and bartenders, as the three most dishonest types of employees. He stated that the phar-macy profession was at a crossroads; clinical pharmacy was neces-sary to the survival of the profession. Gerhard Levy acknowledged that there were two distinct levels of pharmacy practitioners, the indi-viduals who were primarily dispensers and those who provided clini-cal services and were the problem solvers.[38] In 1980, Jere Goyan, who was then commissioner of the FDA, spoke of "the professional chasm between what pharmacists can do and what they actually do."[39] He went on to state that pharmacy's biggest problem was that it was a profession of underachievers, which had not accepted the chal-lenges offered. However, he felt that pharmacists were developing more confidence in themselves, at least in part due to the efforts of schools and colleges of pharmacy. Robert Chalmers in 1980 referred to the Millis Commission's recommendations and stated that although some of them were being implemented, there was "considerable room for additional improvement."[15] Even though the literature from 1979 to 1981 mentioned the problems existing in the pharmacy profession, the commitment to change was also evident. As mentioned previously, the APhA "Policy Statements on the Role of Community Pharmacy" and the "Standards of Practice for the Profession of Pharmacy" provided a road map for the future.[15,34] William Zellmer also stated that hospital pharmacy was committed to providing clinical services. He believed that their implementation on a widespread basis would be the major challenge for the 1980s.[17]

As in previous years, reports during 1980 and 1981 also referred to the division among pharmacy's leaders. One author urged professional pharmacy organizations to unite to promote the profession, regardless of the type of pharmacy practice involved.[40] Apple identified one of the major problems in pharmacy as the division within the pharmacy profession and lack of strong leadership.[20] In fact, he felt the single greatest weakness in the profession was the proliferation of divergent pharmacy organizations and either an absent or irrational overall organizational structure. Although his article pointed out a number of problems existing in the pharmacy profession, Apple ended by stating that the "future holds promise if we only approach it with confidence and responsibility."

An area of discussion in the literature, and some disagreement, related to pharmacy technicians and their role in the profession. The Millis Commission's report referred to the issue of pharmacy technicians as being hotly debated. However, it was predicted that their use would continue to increase and they would become "a recognized part of the system of drug dispensing."[6] The Commission also stated that "The future will not permit the use of the full-trained pharmacist in procedures and tasks that do not require the level of his knowledge and skill."[41] The Commission believed that the colleges of pharmacy should be responsible for the general supervision of technician training and felt that in order for pharmacists to work with them, technicians should be part of the professional education process.[6] Others agreed that the use of technicians should increase.[16,17,42] Oddis felt that pharmacy needed to expand and utilize effectively supportive personnel throughout the profession, particularly in the community setting.[16] In order for this to occur, however, he believed that the community pharmacist must first accept his role as a drug specialist and information provider and not simply as a dispenser of medications. The use of technicians was also said to be increasing to free "pharmacists to use their heads more than their hands."[42] In the hospital setting, it was felt that in order for pharmacy to accomplish its goal of the widespread implementation of clinical services, extensive technician use would be required.[17] It was predicted by the year 2000, a large number of the ASHP membership would represent technicians and technologists, and that they would be legally recognized as associate pharmacists.[40] In contrast to the Millis report, however, the author felt that technicians would continue to be trained in nonacademic or institutionally based programs. In sharp contrast to the call for the enhanced training and use of pharmacy supportive personnel, Apple was strongly against this.[20] He stated that too many pharmacists were being educated and pharmacist unemployment was predicted to increase; by the year 1990, Apple predicted that there could be a 14 percent pharmacist unemployment rate nationwide. Due to this, he was opposed to an increase in technicians. In fact, he stated that "the result predicted by those who wish to increase the training and utilization of pharmacy support personnel is a non sequitur that threatens to sacrifice the economic and professional future of even more pharmacists."[20]

The Study Commission, in addition to advocating the use of technicians to allow pharmacists to assume more patient-oriented responsibilities, believed that technology use would also facilitate the accomplishment of this goal. The Commission felt that pharmacy must become more efficient in its efforts, and that it must take advantage of every opportunity for the use of automation to perform routine, non-professional tasks.[41] The Commission report also indicated that drug information systems would become more complex as available information and the demand for it, as an outgrowth of increased demand for all types of health services, continued to expand. Similarly, a report in 1980 predicted that a computer explosion in pharmacies of all types and sizes would occur by the year 1990.[42] It was stated that some of the large pharmacy chains were developing computer systems that would allow access to patient prescription records by any pharmacist in the chain. Levy indicated "that modern pharmacists must be able to utilize the new tools of information science, particularly those involving retrieval of information."[38] The vision represented in the Commission report more than two decades before is obvious, given the crucial roles (patient profile maintenance, screening for drug interactions and incompatibilities, accessing information databases, delivery of educational programs, etc.) that computers play in our present pharmacy environment.

Another topic of some disagreement in the Study Commission's report involved the role of specialization within the pharmacy profession. The Commission observed that the high degree of specialization that occurred in medicine had brought with it many problems along with benefits.[43] Since the Commission members felt that pharmacy was already a divided profession, they were skeptical of the benefits that would result from further division via specialization. This viewpoint was not consistent with others in pharmacy, however. Lawrence Weaver felt that specialization would occur because it was not possible for a generalist to obtain the skills necessary to practice in all possible areas.[24] He believed that tracking options allowing for career choices would make "the pharmacist more effective and careers more rewarding." Interestingly, he speculated that the ability for specialization to occur within a six-year degree program might still be a goal by the year 1990. Another author, Milton Skolaut, predicted that there would be two practice choices within larger institutions in the future, specialized clinical pharmacy practice or what was termed total pharmacy service practice.[40] He indicated that hospital residency and other training programs should produce pharmacists who could provide for the entire range of patient-oriented services in smaller institutions. These individuals would also help to support the work of the pharmacy specialists. The specialists would function as primary drug and dose prescribers and advisors to physicians.

An issue raised by the Study Commission that is still a problem in the present day relates to the reimbursement of pharmacists for patient care services. The Commission believed that the pharmacist of the future would receive compensation for not only the handling of drug products, but also for the knowledge and skill used in providing the service, whether or not the service actually involved physical delivery of the product.[5] Apple felt that the "clinical pharmacy bubble has to burst," primarily because unless the public was willing to pay for professional pharmacy services, economic realities would be a barrier to the ability of pharmacists to perform nondistributive activities.[20] Goyan agreed and emphasized that pharmacy needs a monetary reward for its nondispensing services, particularly when the pharmacist might spend a significant amount of time in activities that do not result in a product or prescription sale.[39] Even in the present day, the pharmacy profession still has significant progress to make with regard to the Study Commission's vision of appropriate reimbursement for cognitive service provision.

In addition to the changes in the pharmacy education system mentioned previously, the Study Commission believed that interdisciplinary education, education in which pharmacy, medicine, and nursing students learn together and in which other health professionals contribute to the education of pharmacy students, should be strived for.[44] The desirability of such an educational environment was echoed in later publications.[24,38,45] It was stated that when students from different disciplines learn together, enhanced respect for one another's expertise occurs.[24] Levy also called for more closer alignment of pharmacy schools with medical schools and other health professionals.[38] Furthermore, the merger at that time of six colleges of pharmacy with other allied health professions emphasized the importance of increased interdisciplinary awareness and experiences to pharmacy students.[45] Today, although pharmacy students interact frequently with students and professionals from other health care disciplines during experiential rotations, integrated didactic instruction among students from a variety of health profession disciplines is still limited.

The Study Commission also raised the issues of the need to enhance the clinical pharmacy faculty with regard to numbers and training, and an imbalance between the physical and biological sciences, which appeared to be given greater emphasis in the curriculum, and the behavioral and social sciences.[46] These same views were later echoed by other educators.[24,38,47] Significant progress in both the clinical and behavioral areas has since been made in pharmacy education. The Study Commission had also stressed the need for improved communication skills among students and practitioners.[2] As noted in the earlier literature, this need was again espoused by others during 1980.[25,40,47]

CONCLUSION

Change, and the call for change, is inevitable in our society. In his 1976 address, Kinnard stated that

> one gets the feeling that everything has already been said, and I can well imagine a pharmacist back in 1776, or even Galen before that, arguing about the need for a change in pharmacy. We constantly seem to be wandering in the wilderness seeking our true identity.[23]

Likewise, resistance to change by many individuals is also predictable. When change occurs, it often does so in a "piecemeal" manner and not as the result of a well-planned and thought-out approach.

Pharmacists for the Future: The Report of the Study Commission on Pharmacy was truly a landmark for the profession of pharmacy. The report represented a plan for pharmacy education that was well organized, thoughtful, interesting, insightful, and futuristic in its outlook. There is strong evidence in the literature during the first few years following the report's availability that it was read and embraced by many of the pharmacy leaders of the time. In fact, pharmacy as a profession is still grappling today, over twenty years later, with fully implementing several of the excellent recommendations contained within the report. Although not all of the predictions in the report materialized and not all of its recommendations were followed, the Study Commission provided valuable "food for thought" for our profession. As an individual who read the Commission's report in its entirety for the first time, twenty years after its release, the validity of their analyses and recommendations was striking. It was disappointing that, as a student at the time the report was published, I had been unaware of its existence and was not provided with a copy to read and contemplate. Even today, the report should be mandatory reading by pharmacy students in our schools and colleges. Students should be asked to consider both the strengths and weaknesses of the Commission's report. For those recommendations deemed to be of merit that have not yet been implemented widely, they should brainstorm methods by which the goals could be accomplished in all practice sites. Pharmacy schools and colleges should work to ensure that the new entry-level degree programs being developed are actually competency based and produce graduates whose ultimate concern is the patient and his or her well-being. The schools and colleges of pharmacy need to become partners with practitioners and help to resolve the problems that exist still within our profession and the health care delivery system. It is only through this approach that pharmacy as a profession will truly move into the twenty-first century.

NOTES

1. *Pharmacists for the Future: The Report of the Study Commission on Pharmacy* (Health Administration Press, Ann Arbor, MI, 1975), p. 81 [p. 197].*

2. *Pharmacists for the Future: The Report of the Study Commission on Pharmacy* (Health Administration Press, Ann Arbor, MI, 1975), p. 72 [p. 191].

3. *Pharmacists for the Future: The Report of the Study Commission on Pharmacy* (Health Administration Press, Ann Arbor, MI, 1975), pp. 96-98 [pp. 207-209].

4. *Pharmacists for the Future: The Report of the Study Commission on Pharmacy* (Health Administration Press, Ann Arbor, MI, 1975), pp. 101-102 [pp. 210-211].

5. *Pharmacists for the Future: The Report of the Study Commission on Pharmacy* (Health Administration Press, Ann Arbor, MI, 1975), p. 100 [pp. 209-210].

6. *Pharmacists for the Future: The Report of the Study Commission on Pharmacy* (Health Administration Press, Ann Arbor, MI, 1975), pp. 117-118 [p. 221].

7. *Pharmacists for the Future: The Report of the Study Commission on Pharmacy* (Health Administration Press, Ann Arbor, MI, 1975), p. 103 [pp. 211-212].

8. *Pharmacists for the Future: The Report of the Study Commission on Pharmacy* (Health Administration Press, Ann Arbor, MI, 1975), p. 111 [p. 217].

9. D.J. Krigstein, A call for self-discipline, *Am Pharm, NS18,* 19 (1978).

10. D.C. Brodie, "Quo. Vadis," *Am. J. Pharm., 149,* 45 (1977).

11. *Pharmacists for the Future: The Report of the Study Commission on Pharmacy* (Health Administration Press, Ann Arbor, MI, 1975), p. 123 [p. 224].

12. *Pharmacists for the Future: The Report of the Study Commission on Pharmacy* (Health Administration Press, Ann Arbor, MI, 1975), p. 128 [p. 227].

13. H.H. Wolf, Significant issues raised by the Study Commission on Pharmacy report—An educator's perspective, *Am. J. Pharm. Educ., 40,* 445 (1976).

14. *Pharmacists for the Future: The Report of the Study Commission on Pharmacy* (Health Administration Press, Ann Arbor, MI, 1975), p. 93 [p. 205].

15. R.K. Chalmers, Pharmacy education . . . and the future of pharmacy—A plan for action, *Am. Pharm., NS20,* 17 (1980).

16. J.A. Oddis, Pharmacy in the 1980s: A look at patient-oriented pharmacy services, *Milit. Med., 144,* 441 (1979).

17. W.A. Zellmer, Priorities for hospital pharmacy in the 1980s, *Am. J. Hosp. Pharm., 37,* 481 (1980).

18. R.A. Gosselin, The future of pharmacy, *Am. J. Pharm. Educ., 40,* 223 (1976).

19. H.N. Lunan, The challenge and promise of pharmacy in the future, *Hosp. Formul., 11,* 417 (1976).

---

*Bracketed pagination refers to pages in Appendix A.

20. W.S. Apple, Introspection and challenge—Anticipating pharmacy's future, *Am. Pharm., NS21,* 30 (1981).

21. S.M.G. Duffy, Hospital pharmacy: The past, the present, the promise, *Am. J. Hosp. Pharm., 35,* 830 (1978).

22. P. Sacks, The challenges before us, *Am. Pharm., NS18,* 8 (1978).

23. W.J. Kinnard Jr., A sense of identity and a sense of the future—Address of the president-elect, *Am. J. Pharm. Educ., 40,* 438 (1976).

24. L.C. Weaver, Undergraduate education—A look to the future, *Am. Pharm., NS20,* 24 (1980).

25. J.F. Schlegel, Pharmacy education—Looking ahead, *Am. Pharm., NS20,* 18 (1980).

26. E. Cohen, What I expect—What I get: A consumer's view, *Am. Pharm., NS21,* 20 (1981).

27. D.E. Francke, Significant issues raised by the Study Commission on Pharmacy Report—A view from the profession, *Am. J. Pharm. Educ., 40,* 448 (1976).

28. G.F. Archambault, The Millis report and the real world, *Hosp. Formul., 11,* 102 (1976).

29. *Pharmacists for the Future: The Report of the Study Commission on Pharmacy* (Health Administration Press, Ann Arbor, MI, 1975), p. 142 [p. 236].

30. D.C. McLeod, Contribution of clinical pharmacists to patient care, *Am. J. Hosp. Pharm., 33,* 904 (1976).

31. J.W. Miller, Nothing less than unity, *Am. Pharm., NS18,* 12 (1978).

32. M.H. Stolar, National Survey of Hospital Pharmaceutical Services—1978, *Am. J. Hosp. Pharm., 36,* 316 (1979).

33. D.R. Tousignaut, Joint Commission on Accreditation of Hospitals' 1977 Standards for Pharmaceutical Services, *Am. J. Hosp. Pharm., 34,* 943 (1977).

34. S.H. Kalman and J.F. Schlegel, Standards of practice for the profession of pharmacy, *Am. Pharm., NS19,* 22 (1979).

35. H.S. Carlin, Patient accountability—Pharmacists' future, *Am. J. Hosp. Pharm., 35,* 263 (1978).

36. W.A. Zellmer, Reviewing the 1970s: Hospital pharmacy practice, *Am. J. Hosp. Pharm., 36,* 1490 (1979).

37. C.C. Pulliam, The life raft theory, *Am. J. Hosp. Pharm., 35,* 394 (1978).

38. G. Levy, Pharmaceutical education in the future, *Drug Intell. Clin. Pharm., 15,* 590 (1981).

39. J.E. Goyan, A conversation with Commissioner Jere E. Goyan, pharmacist, *Am. Pharm., NS20,* 19 (1980).

40. M.W. Skolaut, Moving toward the 21st century, *Am. J. Hosp. Pharm., 37,* 355 (1980).

41. *Pharmacists for the Future: The Report of the Study Commission on Pharmacy* (Health Administration Press, Ann Arbor, MI, 1975), p. 76 [p. 194].

42. K.A. McGee, Pharmacists will be free to use their heads more than their hands, *Am. Druggist, 49,* 54 (1980).

43. *Pharmacists for the Future: The Report of the Study Commission on Pharmacy* (Health Administration Press, Ann Arbor, MI, 1975), p. 105 [p. 213].

44. *Pharmacists for the Future: The Report of the Study Commission on Pharmacy* (Health Administration Press, Ann Arbor, MI, 1975), p. 130 [p. 229].

45. G.E. Schumacher and J.T. Barr, A new direction for the '80s: The College of Pharmacy and Allied Health Professions, *Am. J. Hosp. Pharm., 37,* 187 (1980).

46. *Pharmacists for the Future: The Report of the Study Commission on Pharmacy* (Health Administration Press, Ann Arbor, MI, 1975), p. 126 [p. 225].

47. B. Stalpes, Learning about the elderly—Closing the gaps, *Am. Pharm., NS20,* 19 (1980).

Chapter 5

Millis Applied: The Minnesota Program

Albert I. Wertheimer

Virtually everyone in North America involved with the practice and science of pharmacy waited with curiosity and great interest to the official release in December 1975 of the final report of the Study Commission on Pharmacy. When the report became available, it was the subject of seminars, retreats, lectures, symposia, study groups, countless task forces, and committees. All of these events were conducted to enable the North American pharmacy community to

1. learn the thoughts and ideas of leaders and thinkers;
2. consider how the findings and recommendations would impact on them and their institutions; and
3. react to the suggested modifications to conventional pharmacy education.

Naturally, there were the skeptics as well, who said that the Study Commission Report, better known as the Millis Commission Report, was just another one of a series of studies that are conducted every few years, spoken about with passion, and then discarded and forgotten shortly thereafter. The skeptics were 100 percent wrong in this situation, probably because they had not done their homework, for had they taken the time or trouble to explore the history of Dr. John S. Millis, they would have learned that this individual always met his goals. There was no secret either as his success was due to hard work, his superior intellect, and his infectious enthusiasm for his projects that spread to those working with him.

The final report was officially titled *Pharmacists for the Future: The Report of the Study Commission on Pharmacy,* and it contained fourteen findings and recommendations.[1] Yet, in addition to these fourteen general concept statements, the report is replete with other findings and recommendations on a more specific basis. For example, in Chapter 11, "The Content of Pharmacy Education," one finds the following passage:

> Pharmacy faculties have a substantial number of well-trained basic scientists in chemistry, medicinal chemistry, pharmacology, and pharmaceutics. They have some truly competent behavioral and social scientists. Some faculties have highly competent pharmacy practitioners, the counterpart of clinical physicians. However, pharmacy faculties have very few members who can be called clinical scientists—people who are equally skilled and trained in a science and in pharmacy practice. . . .
>
> In the view of the Study Commission the greatest contribution which a foundation or governmental agency could make to upgrade pharmacy education, and thereby improve drug services to the public, would be to fund a national program to train a modest number of clinical scientists for pharmacy. One can envision a program to give a hundred or more well-trained pharmacy practitioners the opportunity to acquire deeper scientific knowledge, the skill of rigorous research, and broadened understanding of the management and control of disease. As such persons completed their advanced training they should find important places on pharmacy faculties and fill the void which is so evident.[2]

It was these words which became the seed for discussion at first and then serious planning at the University of Minnesota in Minneapolis during 1976 and 1977. The university has a number of features that made it an ideal venue to attempt implementing such a demonstration/research project. It is fortunate to have a world-class health sciences center which is integrated with outstanding social and behavioral scientists. The city is large enough to supply a diverse patient population for both the clinical facilities and, for interview and survey purposes, the liberal arts and social sciences. The health sciences component contained faculties of medicine, dentistry, nursing, pharmacy, public health, and allied health.

The metropolitan area housed more than twenty hospitals, the headquarters of pharmacy chains, hospital chains, health maintenance organizations, research centers, and high-tech medical device and pharmaceutical manufacturers. In short, it seemed to be an ideal location with more than adequate internal and external resources.

Therefore, in 1977, a decision was made to contact the W. K. Kellogg Foundation for an informal reaction to a proposal to train clinical scientists. This initiative was spearheaded by the two project codirectors, Paul B. Batalden, MD, and Albert I. Wertheimer, PhD. Dr. Batalden, a physician with board certification in pediatrics, was director of a prepaid group practice plan, a faculty member in the School of Medicine, and a past director of a unit of the U.S. Public Health Service. Dr. Wertheimer was a professor and director of graduate studies in social and administrative pharmacy at the School of Pharmacy and a managed care consultant.

Drs. Batalden and Wertheimer took the Commission's recommendation Number 10 that "support be sought for a program to train a modest number of clinical scientists for pharmacy education" and, with the marvelous backing of then Minnesota Pharmacy Dean Lawrence C. Weaver, received endorsement from the entire College of Pharmacy faculty. Dean Weaver later wrote,

> It was immediately apparent that guidance and perspective from other sources would be valuable to the success of the project. The natural first step was to ask Dr. Millis to chair an advisory group. He agreed to do so, and we were quite pleased because he knew the complete workings of the original Study Commission and was knowledgeable in this realm, in pharmacy as well as in other professions. A physicist by education and subsequently a medical educator, university chancellor and Director of the National Fund for Medical Education, Dr. Millis was widely regarded as one of the most brilliant and insightful thinkers of the day.[3]

The remainder of the advisory group was assembled. Each member was selected for his personal traits, accomplishments, and affiliations. Dr. Leighton (Lee) Cluff, then president of the Robert Wood Johnson Foundation of Princeton, New Jersey, was invited, as were Dr. Lawrence Weaver, dean of the College of Pharmacy; Mr. Jerome Halperin, then acting director of the Bureau of Drugs of the Food and Drug Administration, and later president of the U.S. Pharmacopoeia; Mr. Lawrence C. Hoff, president of the Upjohn Company; and Dr.

Gerald Schumacher of Northeastern University School of Pharmacy. Drs. Wertheimer and Bataldem completed the group.

A goal was established, to produce clinical scientists in pharmacy, to give well-trained pharmacy practitioners the opportunity to acquire deeper scientific knowledge, the skills of rigorous research, and broadened understanding of management and control of disease. It was expected that the graduates would fill important places on pharmacy faculties and leadership positions in a variety of potential careers in recognized and unrecognized areas related to pharmacy.[4]

Funding from the Kellogg Foundation began in 1979 with a grant of $846,600. Supplemental amounts were added so that by 1989 slightly over $1 million was provided in total.

University of Minnesota Kellogg Pharmaceutical Clinical Scientist fellows were expected to pursue a course of study leading to the receipt of a PhD in social and administrative pharmacy within a span of thirty-six months. Fellows had individually customized courses of study planned for them following extensive discussions with their advisors. The anticipation at the outset of the program was that the fellows would proceed first through a series of required core courses where they would exercise personal inclinations by selecting one or two tracks of specialized study. The two available tracks were

1. Clinical Practice Administration
2. Research in Clinical Practice

Core courses for both tracks included legislative control (covering the historical development and social and economic causes and consequences of drug and health legislation), pharmaceutical economics, drug marketing, social and behavioral aspects of pharmacy practice, research design, statistics, data processing, medical sociology, and required monthly seminars and weekly departmental seminars throughout the duration of a fellow's studies.[5]

Students in Track 1 added the following course work to the core requirements: accounting, industrial relations, finance, psychology of advertising, elements of public health, public health administration, health education, epidemiology, vital statistics, management, management information systems, human resources in health services organizations, long-term care administration, and other subjects/disciplines depending upon the needs and goals of that individual.

Track 2 fellows studied the following in addition to the core elements: program evaluation, advanced research methods, biostatistics, principles of measurement, behavioral analysis, multivariate analysis, research planning, aging, and clinical trials.

Recruitment was achieved through advertisements and press releases sent to major pharmacy organizations, schools of pharmacy, local societies, and publications such as newsletters and journals. A poster with return postcards was also distributed widely. The candidates were asked to complete the standard University of Minnesota graduate school admission application materials, a departmental supplementary application form, and a special fellowship form requesting information on employment history, professional, service, or community-related activities, professional affiliations, and professional or scientific publications and presentations. In addition, a writing sample was requested, and answers to the following questions were called for:

1. At this time, what areas of investigation do you believe would hold the most interest for you as a pharmaceutical clinical scientist?
2. In what ways do you believe your professional experience to date will relate to your preparation and future performance as a pharmaceutical clinical scientist?
3. What roles and needs for your services as a pharmaceutical clinical scientist do you envision in academic, health care delivery and/or research environments?
4. Under what circumstances and by what methods have you most successfully exercised leadership?
5. What do you believe have been your most important (a) personal and (b) professional accomplishments?
6. Do you believe that your prior academic performance is representative of your abilities? If your answer is no, please explain.
7. In your view, why should you be admitted to this program, and what strengths will you bring to it?

When application forms were received, an applicant evaluation process was initiated. Core faculty members were asked to evaluate the applications and to employ a standardized scoring system adopted from the one used by the Markle Foundation Scholars Program which was based upon modifications to the British Foreign Service application forms. (It was Dr. Millis who knew of these programs, application forms, etc.) Promising applicants were invited for an in-person interview.

It is fair to say that there probably was not a single aspect of the program where Dr. Millis did not make enormous contributions. His thoughts and ideas in the conceptualization process and concurrent early phases proved to all of us that this man was a one-in-a-million. He had ideas, suggestions, and cautions from many years of diverse experience. When we did not know where to turn for something, he always had an idea or two, and to be sure, just mentioning his name when we contacted perfect strangers brought us instant acceptance and help. In fact, in nearly a decade of work with this activity, we never ran into anyone who had a negative thought or who harbored any bad feelings toward this wonderful man. With us, he freely shared his ideas, thoughts, suggestions, and the lessons he had learned the hard way from previous experience. He shared his contacts, and as a fringe benefit he shared his outstanding sense of humor and observations on daily events, news of the day, or whatever happened to tickle his fancy at that point in time.

It was recognized from the very beginning that clinical scholars could be produced by a combination of pharmacology and psychology, or of pharmaceutics and sociology, or of pathology and public health and with countless combinations of inputs from any one of the thousands of universities in the United States alone. We envisioned our graduates to be broader thinkers than clinicians alone or researchers alone. Hopefully, they would have the tools to objectively assess situations and then have the knowledge, understanding, and motivation to do something about situations that are less than ideal. These are change agents in no uncertain terms. In fact, one of the most common phrases from Dr. Millis was the term "divine discontent." He urged us to instill a divine discontent in the fellows, to create change agents who are prepared to see situations in their totality and know how the political, economic, and legislative domains function so that they can be employed to "get things done."

Of the fifteen candidates who accepted fellowships, fourteen completed the course work, and to date, thirteen of those fourteen have completed their PhD requirements and are employed in related areas:

Nicholas Bartone   MaryKay Oleen
Jon Clouse   Tom Rector
Jack Fincham   Leonard Rosenberg
Brian Isetts   Bernard Sorofman
Ralph Kalies   Richard Spivey
Lucinda Maine   Julie Zito
Robert Nelson

Meetings were held on an annual basis for several years after the completion of the active fellowship program to provide the fellows an opportunity to exchange experiences and to learn from one another's travails. Clearly, the fellows were prepared to become active change agents, and since there is always resistance to change, it was hoped that the fellows might profit from learning which strategies worked for their classmates and which methodologies failed.

Today, there is no Kellogg Pharmaceutical Clinical Scientist program at the university or elsewhere. This is not seen as a failure, but rather as a recognition that the Study Commission's recommendation was quite accurate. A small number of such persons, if the concept was accurate, could start through a cadre effort an important new era in pharmacy education and later in practice. A costly, labor-intensive program such as the one described herein could not be sustained on an ongoing basis, nor should that be an objective. The cost for preparing the thirteen successful fellows was nearly $100,000 (in 1980 dollars) each.

Whether the program succeeded will have to be determined in the future when a clearer picture evolves as to the impact of this brave band of pioneer change agents. Perhaps the best way to make any type of objective assessment is to review the Study Commission recommendation and then balance it against what we do know today. The full citation of recommendation Number 10 follows:

> It is the opinion of the Study Commission that the greatest weakness of the schools of pharmacy is a lack of an adequate number of clinical scientists who can relate their specialized scientific knowledge to the development of the practice skills required to provide effective, efficient and needed patient services. The Study Commission recommends that support be sought for a program to train a modest number of clinical scientists for pharmacy education.

Much more can be said about the endeavor at Minnesota, but that has already been done through reports to the Kellogg Foundation, several journal articles, newsletters, and a single issue of the *Journal of Pharmacy Teaching* (vol. 1, #2, 1990) entirely devoted to a complete report on the Minnesota Kellogg Pharmaceutical Clinical Scientist program.

What remains is to add some previously unpublished insight into the involvement and contributions of one Dr. John S. Millis. All of us who worked on the program came to have the fondest feelings and unlimited respect for this giant of a scholar. To be honest, we suspected and later knew that he was proud to be associated with the implementation of his intellectual concept. Surely, in any policy discussion, he could have had his way, but amazingly, it never came to that. He usually prevailed because of the depth of thought in his stance or argument. After learning more facts, or hearing an opposing view, it was not uncommon for him to modify or even slightly improve his original idea or proposal. While his spirit and enthusiasm were always with us, in fact, Dr. Millis visited Minneapolis only two or three times per year to meet with the fellows and staff for planning or review sessions, nearly always accompanied by Mrs. Millis.

When I think back to 1978-1980 and the informal planning sessions with Dr. Millis (who asked us to call him Jack), there is one overwhelming mental image that presents itself. The same chain of events I picture in various settings. The sequence began with something being said by another person. Jack Millis's hand would go onto his chin and there would be silence for about ten to fifteen seconds. This was followed by a little twinkle of a smile and then we heard some eloquently phrased statement that politely told us again and again that there was a simple way to accomplish something or another by just doing X and Y. When Jack was not present, we found ourselves working to make certain that he would not be disappointed in us when he next learned about our latest idea or program feature. He was like a big brother, protecting us from our own shortcomings and lack of experience. I cannot recall him ever raising his voice, as that was not his style. Intellectual prowess wins out over bullies and demagogues, I'm sure he believed. In fact, even when we recognized later, with his guidance, that we had erred, it was presented in such a way that one could begin to see his own mistake.

It would be true to say that he never failed to amaze us. About a year before his death, he decided to read and teach himself molecular biology. When asked why, he calmly reported that it was becoming an important discipline and that he did not know very much about it and therefore felt an obligation or inner need to learn about this important topic. Dr. Millis comes as close as anyone I have ever known, or actually, closer, to what I understand is a renaissance man. And for that matter, I don't expect to have to change that statement during the rest of my lifetime.

Humor was the man's other contribution to the program. During a tense time, we heard an anecdote that was funny, relevant, and most often contained a valuable parable for us to consider. I still remember asking what it felt like to have a university administration or classroom building named in his honor and he replied that he was much more enthusiastic about the women's dormitory named after him.

In an article put together nearly a decade ago, I reconstructed the words, written and oral, of Dr. Millis's more than five years of active participation in the program at the University of Minnesota. Some of his thoughts and suggestions were given privately to Dr. Batalden and myself, and others were given in presentations or correspondence. In all of these exchanges, his wit and intelligence showed through clearly. Any report of the Minnesota Program would be incomplete without incorporating these insights (Addendum).

Personally speaking, I will always owe a massive debt of gratitude to this man. The 1975 recommendation was the catalyst for an exciting decade of my professional life in which I learned a great deal, had the opportunity to work with giants, and, within a group effort, made what I truly hope will be a contribution to pharmacy education and practice for a long time to come. In retrospect, there was a reasonable probability that the Kellogg Foundation might not have chosen to invest a great deal of money in this comparative youngster were Dr. Millis not so intimately involved. He provided us his time, patience (not always deserved), keen insight, knowledge, and experience. For all of this I will be forever grateful and, simultaneously, proud and honored that I count myself a fortunate person to have worked with Dr. John S. Millis.

NOTES

1. *Pharmacists for the Future: The Report of the Study Commission on Pharmacy* (Health Administration Press, Ann Arbor, MI, 1975).

2. *Pharmacists for the Future: The Report of the Study Commission on Pharmacy* (Health Administration Press, Ann Arbor, MI, 1975), pp. 124-125 [pp. 224-225].*

3. L.C. Weaver, The Kellogg Pharmaceutical Clinical Scientist Program: History and development, *J. Pharm. Teach., 1,* 37 (1990).

4. A.I. Wertheimer and P.B. Batalden, Introduction, *J. Pharm. Teach., 1,* 5 (1990).

5. A.I. Wertheimer, The Kellogg Pharmaceutical Clinical Scientist Program: Nuts and bolts, *J. Pharm. Teach., 1,* 20 (1990).

*Bracketed pagination refers to pages in Appendix A.

Addendum

Thoughts for the Kellogg Pharmaceutical Clinical Scientist Program

John S. Millis

My thoughts on the Kellogg Pharmaceutical Clinical Scientist Program arise from what I have observed in the last twenty to twenty-five years as an outsider in the health professions, looking at and sometimes being asked to comment on and to help within the fields of medicine, dentistry, nursing, pharmacy, and nutrition. I have found it necessary to try to create for myself a conceptual model of what I am observing, to understand it in the broad picture, and to try to relate all that I observe and all the conclusions I reach to that model.

The Study Commission on Pharmacy was a remarkable experience for me; after two years we were thinking almost as one individual. The most obvious criticism of the present health care system was its capacity for generating a reverse flow of knowledge from the point of experience and understanding back toward the preceding parts of the system. It became evident in studying pharmacy that this was the most severe deficit—and it was nowhere nearly as pronounced in the field of medicine. The one thing that flows through the system in pharmacy is products. Knowledge gets thrown in the wastebasket (with the exception of reporting adverse reactions). No one in pharmacy is in charge of feedback, and this must be accomplished with people; hence, the concept of the clinical scientist.

This article, originally published in the *Journal of Pharmacy Teaching* 1(2):71-82, was compiled from the speeches Dr. Millis gave to the project staff and students over a period of several years. Dr. Millis was an internationally recognized physicist who became a medical educator. At the time of his recent death, he was chancellor emeritus of Case Western Reserve University in Cleveland, Ohio.

Historically, the starting point of knowledge in the system we call health care has been the biomedical sciences—good old trusty subjects called anatomy, pathology, physiology, pharmacology, and biochemistry. But what has happened is that inexorably the width of this spectrum has been increasing. That is, the physician/scholar has found something in physics that is important to the doctor. The pharmacist has found something in behavioral psychology or social psychology and cultural anthropology that is relevant to pharmacy. How people react to the pharmacist and drugs is not only a personal experience but also a group experience—it is a cultural, a societal, phenomenon. We've known right along that economics has something to do with it. Suddenly, we find out that to serve society we not only have to give health care that is effective, but we also have to give health care that is efficient. Cost containment is now the motto of every professional. It has to be. We also found out that the communication sciences are important, and we found out that the managerial sciences are very, very relevant. Suddenly we're faced with the fact that rather than dealing with a rather narrow spectrum for the acquisition of knowledge, we have an entire spectrum involving all of these areas.

I want to draw some maps so that you know where I am in the hope that you will be with me and we won't be talking off and against each other. First, I want to tell you that there is a tried and true method I always use, a set of steps. I always want to get from here to there in an orderly process if there is to be a chance of any final success.

A number of times I have been asked to think about certain problems in the field of medicine—graduate education, for instance, or, more recently, evaluation of the national boards—or nursing, where I have worked over several years, or pharmacy. Over the years it has occurred to me that there is a pattern, a similarity, a parallelism, whether one is working in genetics or in medicine or in nursing or in pharmacy, that allows one to design a generic diagram that describes the system.

This model makes an assumption, which you may or may not challenge. For me, it has worked extremely well—better than any model I have seen. It conceives of the system we call the health care system not as a service system but as a knowledge system, one of the products of which is various kinds of care offered to the public and to the individual patient. In this, perhaps, it resembles the communication system, which is a knowledge system that produces means of communication called telephones, satellites, telegraphs, or something of that sort. But this system, to me, is a very interesting knowledge system that produces a socially and individually useful service that we call health care.

Now, in that system there are four very clear parts. I say this, and I want you to remember it, because if you read the standard literature and listen to the usual conversation, you find that people deal with the health care system in tripart imagery. We too frequently have thought of medicine in terms of a three-legged stool called research, education, and patient care, and every dean bragged that he had a three-legged stool on which the legs were all of equal length and therefore it was stable and was to be greatly admired. But for me, this system is not one of three legs or three parts, sometimes related, sometimes not related. Rather, it is a remarkably integrated, rational system if one looks at it not as a service or research system or educational system or discipline, but as a knowledge system in which all these are elements. It's a four-part system—a clear, logical, and, fortunately, rational system of four parts.

The first of these four parts is knowledge acquisition. This is familiar—research, if you will. It's the acquisition of knowledge. I use the word "acquisition" because it covers at least two different concepts: the initial discovery of knowledge and the simple identification of knowledge in a field that one never before looked at and that one suddenly finds relevant. For example, much of the knowledge that is now in the discipline called biophysics has been a part of physics knowledge for quite a long time. Only recently did we discover that that knowledge was relevant to biology and, therefore, to the biomedical art. This is also true in other disciplines, such as sociology, psychology, economics, philosophy and ethics, communication theory, organizational management, and so forth. So, acquisition has two parts: it may be the original discoveries that one thinks of as pure research—at the bench, for example, when one finds a new enzyme or decodes RNA or DNA. There also is the identification—the recognition—of knowledge that suddenly has become relevant, although it did not seem so in the past.

What struck me immediately about pharmacy was that it draws its knowledge from the entire spectrum more than any other field in the health science system. Our tendency in thinking about pharmacy is to focus on the product. But drugs alone are essentially powerless. What we're trying to get is drugs and the knowledge that is germane to using them effectively. Pharmacy needs knowledge about behavior, communication, and economics. The hurdle that has tripped many people is not realizing that the pharmacist must excel in all of these disciplines. Pharmacists are on the firing point when it comes to knowledge utilization.

Second, there is the process of knowledge translation. Some people call that clinical research. It is the step by which one turns knowledge into a skill—surgical, for instance, or diagnostic, or therapeutic. Or one may turn a part of the knowledge into a product, such as a drug or a device like a pacemaker or an artificial kidney. It's the step in which this knowledge, either discovered through research or borrowed from some existing discipline, is then translated into skill, technology, and product. There is a translation in the art, skill, technique, technology, product, or device. The important point here is that in this process only a part of the knowledge acquired is turned into a product or skill. There is a very substantial and oft-neglected remainder of knowledge that is not encapsulated in a surgical procedure or a drug or a device. There is knowledge about that drug, its activities, its kinetics, its adverse reactions, and its interactions. So we come now from knowledge to the translation of some parts of that knowledge into skills, technologies, techniques, or products.

The third step is knowledge transmission, the step in which we transmit the knowledge, the skills, the technology, the product, into new forms. We academicians are very prone to think this is our bailiwick and that we do the whole thing, that we take all of this knowledge—our knowledge about these devices and these skills and technological developments (the second step, translation)—and transmit it by the education of a physician or a pharmacist, a nurse or a clinical psychologist. But there are a lot of other parts to transmission. There is the formal education of a professional, but there is also communication through the mass media; through the formal educational process, such as health courses in grade schools; through learned journals and popular journals; through TV; and through radio. In this step there is also the distribution of all these products and devices. In pharmacy, this is very important because it is the distribution as well as the manufacture of the products. Professional education is only one part of this transmission. There are many other parts.

Finally, there is knowledge utilization—clinical, if you wish to use that word. This is the point where this knowledge and these devices, these skills, and these technologies are used by professionals called physicians, pharmacists, nurses, etc. They are also used by the people called patients and by organized society in the form of government. That would be the fields of public health and environmental health, where society gets organized via its institutions to use that knowledge at this particular stage. This is the point where the service occurs. This is the point at which the service becomes a visible product.

But there are other parts. There is the recognition of the relevance of already-known knowledge, which is equally important in the acquisition process. All of a sudden, the medics found knowledge that has been around for a long time in my field of physics that was relevant to the process of understanding disease and learned something about it. Pharmacy has discovered knowledge in the field of management sciences, communication, and in the behavioral sciences of psychology and anthropology, and so forth, that is relevant to pharmacy. You didn't have to go back to the bench, so to speak, and get those de novo. I use acquisition, therefore, for the more familiar term of research, which is the discovery of heretofore unknown data, ideas, and theories, as well as the identification of already discovered knowledge that suddenly becomes relevant.

That's the system. It has the asset, it seems to me, that it is logical. It's one of the most beautifully organized, most rational systems I know of in our society. But it is not rational when looked upon as a service system. It is rational only when looked upon as a knowledge system. It has some very serious limitations. One of the most obvious characteristics is that the natural—I shall call it gravitational—flow from the input point to the output point is down. By the nature of the process, the direction is always downward. Knowledge goes from acquisition through translation through transmission to utilization. It's almost a one-way system. It is not a system in which what one has learned at the utilization point comes back into the translation point. There are no natural, inherent, automatic mechanisms in this system for feedback. It is almost a unilateral system. The question is, how do we get what we learn at the utilization—the clinical—stage to affect what it is we look for in our knowledge acquisition or translation systems so that we modify the educational enterprise or other parts of the transmission system to make the system more effective in terms of the actual patient and societal outcome?

Remembering that there are a number of parallel systems called medicine, pharmacy, dentistry, and so forth, the other fault that one could attribute to this system is that there is no automatic system by which the knowledge that comes out of pharmacy gets translated into the medical system and vice versa. Very little comes out of nursing that anybody pays attention to in the medical world, and this is another problem. Essentially, what we must do for society as a whole and as individual patients is to try to give this system an agency that will provide feedback from the utilization point back into the acquisition point, the translation point, or the transmission point.

Third, the most obvious, the most serious, flaw in the system is this lack of a main feedback or a number of feedback systems. It was this conclusion that led the Study Commission on Pharmacy to ask itself, "If we recognize this and if it is an important matter in terms of pharmacy, what suggestions do we have to induce at least one, if not several, feedback mechanisms in this system to improve it as a whole, to make the facts that can be learned at the utilization stage begin to affect the acquisition step, the translation step, and the transmission step?" Our conclusion was that one has to do it with people. We could not conceive of any protocol or sophisticated computer that would suffice: it required people. Think of the kind of person who would be described as polyvalent, having several powers, competencies, capacities. This person could participate actively and competently at the utilization stage. This person could be a clinician who could talk to other clinicians. He would have the language, the experience, the status, the investment of stature, the appropriate position, and he could, at the same time, be useful and contributory at the acquisition stage as a scholar. We call him a clinical scientist. We were tempted to use "artist-scientist" or "scientist-artist" or something because we were dealing with the world of knowing—science—and the world of doing—art. This is a clinical practitioner and scientist.

We were afraid people would take that word "scientist" to mean a man studying mathematics, physics, biochemistry, and subjects of this sort—the hard sciences. We're using the word "scientist" in its generic context, which is simply a knower, a person who deals with knowledge, its discovery and utilization, and its interpretation and organization. That's the meaning of scientist. And "clinical," again, is a slippery word. It comes from the Greek word "klinikos," to lie down. Obviously, a first clinical instruction of medical students was on horizontal patients, and therefore it was a clinical experience. We have now used it in such a way as to change its meaning. It does mean "doing," and, therefore, it's a knowledgeable doer, a doing scholar, a clinical scholar. This is the concept: a person who would be able to know, communicate, participate, be active, contribute as a knower and a doer, the clinical scholar.

Well, what can we do about it? I've been trying to answer the question "why?" Now the question is, "Where do we try to go?" We have had, historically, individuals working in the system who lived and worked in at least two of these steps. For many years we have had the clinical professor who takes care of patients and also teaches medical students. We have the clinical instructor in dentistry, the clinical instructor in nursing, the clinical instructor in pharmacy. So, we are familiar with people who work in both the utilization and the transmission phases. We've also been familiar with people who have worked both at the research bench and on the faculty of a medical school or school of pharmacy, or something of this sort, who have combined the acquisition of knowledge with the transmission of knowledge in the education of professional students. Although this has provided a feedback mechanism between two adjacent steps, it has not provided feedback between the first step and the last step, or, for that matter, between the second and the last steps. The only attempt to do this was the Markle Scholar Program, which attempted to produce the clinical scientist in medicine, the practicing physician who could hold his own in physiological research, biochemistry, or pharmacology, etc. We have some of those people in the system, and I think that they've had a tremendous impact on medical education in the last two, perhaps the last three, decades.

Immediately, everybody says, "all right, clinical scholar." The image comes right back to what we have seen in medicine, where one takes an internist or a pediatrician and gives that person the opportunity to work in a laboratory of physiology or neurobiology or something of that sort, and he becomes at least a competent bench scientist at the same time he is having actual contact with real, perplexing patients with problems. The natural thought is that, following that model, one would try to take a competent practitioner of pharmacy and put him into a department of pharmacology, physiology, biophysics, immunology, or endocrinology and let him become a bench scientist there to hold his own with the PhD of those fields or with those few MDs/PhDs.

What is happening here is not what one would call the instinctive idea of the "doer-knower"—that is, the clinical scientist. By "clinical," I mean "doing." And science in the way I use "scientist" is the generic word meaning "all of knowledge." Rather than having only the opportunity of the basic biomedical sciences, it is the opportunity of coupling the practice of pharmacy with scholarship in the behavioral, economic, and social sciences. This is the recognition of two ideas. One is the recognition of the need for an individual who will be the feedback mechanism to make this system better. Knowledge gained here (at the utilization point) comes back and is recycled to the system through the ever-increasingly important effectiveness, economy, and efficiency of the system in terms of what it actually does for people individually and collectively. The other is recognition of the fact that an awful lot of knowledge already existing or being discovered now, out here in this part of the spectrum that we call behavioral, social, organizational, and administrative sciences, is relevant to this whole process of serving mankind. So much for the concept of the clinical scholar—the knower and doer. We get too much tied up in the words scientist and clinical. It's the knower and the doer.

We see the individual I've described serving as a catalyst within this system, actually learning from his practice, being able to make judgments, to find new understanding and insight that will be useful at the acquisition stage, the translation stage, and the transmission stage. How is he to make these contributions? Well, obviously, in our universities there are all kinds of people. They observe the physician who is running the hospitals, observe the inadequacies in the knowledge, the skill, the technology, and then they go back to the technology in genetics or pharmacology. There are people who are called clinical pharmacologists who do pretty good work at the bench in the department of pharmacology and remarkably good work at the bedside treating patients. I have used the word polyvalent for this concept, but there are limitations on that word. There is a polyvalent assumption: that the clinical scientist can be infinitely poly. This is not true. As a clinician, he will have to confine himself to one particular area. I think one has to look at the spectrum of disciplines that are reasonably relevant to the health science system concerned. The best a clinical scientist could do would be to take hunks out of that system and become polyvalent in a chosen area. What we are talking about is multidisciplinary. Let's stop talking about "interdisciplinary," which means falling between the cracks. This is the only base upon which you could create the polyvalent scientist. By poly, I mean bipoly or tripoly—I don't mean polyvalent. A clinician has a limited area of expertise. He can't have too broad a disciplinary base without becoming a dilettante. We're not going to have a man practicing internal medicine, pediatrics, pharmacy, and radiology.

I would also comment on the process of creating clinical scientists. This is a very important consideration. The process by which people become able to do something is the process which we normally call training. The process by which one becomes a scholar is education. We frequently use these two words interchangeably, saying "education and training" or "education or training." This seems to indicate that they are quite the same thing. They are really fundamentally very different. One of the processes is to know; the other is to do, through knowing of course, but the outcome is doing, doing well and reliably. So there's a process that has to be used to produce the clinical scientist that we're talking about, which comes about through both education and training. When I have said this to other people, they have said to me, "Well, what's the difference?" One of my teachers, Albert A. Michelson, said that training was the process by which the master would raise the apprentice to his level of skill and capacity, but education was the process by which the teacher lifted the scholar to his shoulders so he might stand thereon and go beyond. For me, there is a very real, meaningful difference between those two processes.

Other people through the years have had problems when they were faced with the necessity of both educating and training. I think graduate medical education is our very best example. It is difficult in those years of the residency to continue the process of learning as knowing and the process of being able to do when applying the skills of doing. It was for this reason that the Commission on Medical Education strongly recommended that the university take much more responsibility for graduate medical education than it has in the past to produce individuals who are both trained and educated. This is relevant to the kind of situation you have here. This program is a partnership of the university and a number of excellent clinical institutions drawing a fine line between scholarship and services. And they are two different environments. They have two different scopes or purposes; they have two different modes of operation. You have to provide that symbiosis in which the partnership of these two agencies is such that the individuals who are responsible for the clinical scientists' futures will have the opportunity both to teach in the scholarly sense and to train in terms of clinical expertise, competence, and reliability, and this may give you some problems every now and then. But you will not be able to pull apart and separate these parts in terms of your understanding and commitment to this single challenge.

One way I expect clinical scientists to have an impact on the profession is by becoming faculty members at schools of pharmacy. Hopefully, a clinical scientist would not be too much of a gadfly to wear out his welcome soon. There are some models for this, in fact. The Markle Scholars have had an influence on the medical schools of this country. I can see the clinical scientists having a substantial effect in key positions in the health care system. Perhaps it is too much to hope that they might have some cataclysmic effect by going to DHEW or other organizations of that nature, but one can hope. They might have quite an impact in HMOs. I can think of a number of different environments where a catalyst is needed and could be effective. I don't know whether a clinical scientist could have much effect in a pharmaceutical association, such as the Association of Pharmaceutical Manufacturers.

You've got to understand that this is, in a very real sense, a venture of faith. We aren't quite sure where the clinical scientists are going or that when they get there they're going to have done anything very important. On the other hand, you do have a conviction, I hope, that this is a very important undertaking, and nobody can give you an assurance of success. I use the expression "divine discontent." In my observation, the one thing that makes a university go is that it has a few people who are divinely discontented with the status quo: "We can turn out better doctors than we have been, . . . engineers . . . you name it, and let's do it." In a sense, you're trying to manipulate that quality of divine discontent. I'm not talking about the people who say, "*They* ought to make a better so-and-so" but about the people who say, "*We* can do this better" and then go and do it. What I'm urging here, and what I think I feel in some of you, is a certain amount of divine discontent. I use the words "venture" and "faith" because there is no certainty about this, but there's hope and there's faith that it is worth doing and that it can be done well. I use the words "divine discontent" to indicate something that is rather unusual in the human personality, but it is a very powerful force.

In response to the argument that the world doesn't need anyone as highly trained as the clinical scientist, I would say that the human race could probably last several more millennia without any more creative thought, but I don't think the Lord wants it that way. We have minds to use. We have very few people who think both theoretically and practically. There is a great gap in pharmacy between the bench scientist and those who have to deal with medication. Mankind has not been very astute in seeing the need for a person to bridge this gap. We must recognize that we're not training a cadre of people for a specific job. We are trying to get a few people into the system with the ability to see and observe in the hope that we get a few who can improvise, improve, and expand, who can point out better ways to do things.

Now this is the image, pure and simple, of the clinical scholar in pharmacy that the Study Commission has proposed and that has found fertile ground in this institution. It might be possible to take an adequately educated, trained, and experienced pharmacist who has been on the firing line in the practice of pharmacy and to so deepen and widen his knowledge, his horizons, and his interests that he would be one of the feedback groups in this system, taking what we observe and learn in the utilization phase back into the level of acquisition or translation.

My concept is that we could provide the necessary feedback into the system if we could train a relatively limited number of individuals to be polyvalent—knowers and doers of these businesses that lead to a command of the language and education and understanding. If you could do this, you might be able to affect the system in a very important and useful way, to make it much more reflexive and much more efficient, and to improve the cost-benefit ratio that is important to the people of the United States who pay the bills.

In recruiting candidates, look for excitement about and commitment to pharmacy, a well-organized and disciplined mind, a capacity for work, and an evangelical spirit; look for formulators and communicators. You cannot describe a clinical scientist in terms of a job. You have to describe the individual, but you must recognize potential problems as well.

What I have been trying to tell you is where I think you ought to be trying to go and, more importantly, why. This is novel not only in terms of the concept of the clinical scientist, but also in the field of pharmacy. It's not new in the field of medicine, but it is new in the area of knowledge that you're trying to look at in order to improve the utilization of pharmacy knowledge for the benefit of the patients as individuals and for society as a whole.

So I get excited about this project. I'm trying to infect you with the same kind of excitement. You're on a double frontier. You're in three-dimensional space. I think you're moving out in the two-dimensional space of industry, but you're also moving out in the three-dimensional space of the totality of health care in the several systems.

Postscript

The Millis Commission—was it the mother or the midwife of changes in the profession after 1976—or was it simply a voyeur, watching from afar? Was it a success or a failure? How will we assess the impact of the Commission and separate it from other ongoing influences? While these are serious and important questions, they may not be the right questions.

At the very least, the Millis Commission represents a turning point for the profession of pharmacy. Analogous to the work of Copernicus in the mid-1500s, who hypothesized that the planets revolved around the sun rather than around earth, the Commission served as a citizens' committee and therefore above the vested interests of the profession. As such, it called for a move from a product-centered to a patient-centered profession. The Commission served to provide the introspection of a maturing profession which was looking to understand the needs of the society it served rather than just the needs of the profession that it was examining.

John S. Millis responded to the question of success and I, for one, am willing to listen to his voice as we continue to watch, and facilitate, the profession's move closer to the patient.

> The vast majority of human beings (perhaps ninety or ninety-five percent) want solutions and rarely are interested in problems and understanding them. They pay no attention to the lessons of history and they do not understand them if they are brought to their attention. They have not accepted the wisdom encapsulated in the Principal Principle—"The cause of most of our problems is solutions."
>
> The Study Commission began at the logical end of its study with conceptualization and spent most of its time there. We did work hard on the next step of logic, namely, process. We finally got to the third step of logical analysis, namely, mechanism; but we spent little or no time on nuts and bolts. To most human beings this is an alien behavior for they much prefer to talk about

nuts and bolts and avoid the intellectual labor of conceptualization. Hence, they are quick to criticize the absence of extensive discussion of details (nuts and bolts) without any pause to ask the question whether what is needed is rivets or spot welds and not nuts and bolts at all.

We shall not know for at least ten years whether our Report is good or bad. If by 1986 pharmacy education has changed so as to produce more effective, more knowledgeable, more skillful pharmacists; if by 1990 some of the unmet needs in drug related health services are met; if by 1990 pharmacists and physicians are working closely together to serve patients so that there is a rational drug therapy in this country; if by 1995 there is a free flow of drug information to pharmacists, physicians, nurses and the public—then we must say the Report was good. If none of these things happen, then we must say we failed as do the great majority of commissions.[1]

NOTE

1. J. Millis, "Letter to Chalmers, May 4, 1976" (1DD9, Box 42, Case Western Reserve University Archives), 4 pp.

Appendix A

Pharmacists for the Future: The Report of the Study Commission on Pharmacy

Commissioned by
The American Association of Colleges of Pharmacy
1975

Health Administration Press
Ann Arbor

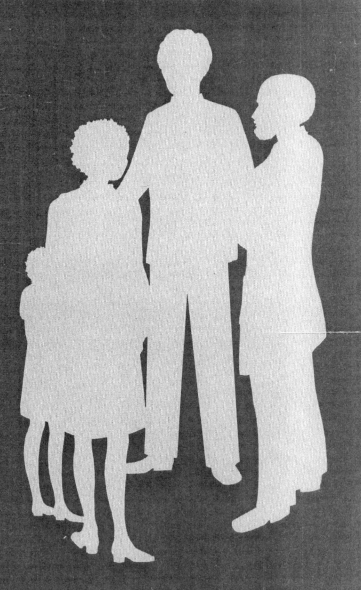

PHARMACISTS FOR THE FUTURE

CONTENTS

MEMBERSHIP OF THE STUDY COMMISSION
ON PHARMACY

John A. Biles, PhD
Dean, School of Pharmacy
University of Southern California
Los Angeles, California

Robert K. Chalmers, PhD
Associate Dean and Professor of Clinical Pharmacy
School of Pharmacy and Pharmacal Sciences
Purdue University
West Lafayette, Indiana

Leighton E. Cluff, MD
Professor and Chairman
Department of Medicine
College of Medicine
University of Florida
Gainesville, Florida

Henry F. DeBoest,* BS
Former Vice President, Corporate Affairs
Eli Lilly and Company
Indianapolis, Indiana

Bryce Douglas, PhD
Vice President, Research and Development
Smith Kline & French Laboratories
Philadelphia, Pennsylvania

Jan Koch-Weser, MD
Associate Professor of Pharmacology
Harvard Medical School and Chief of Clinical Pharmacology Unit
Massachusetts General Hospital
Boston, Massachusetts

John S. Millis, PhD, Chairman
Chairman, National Fund for Medical Education
and Chancellor Emeritus
Case Western Reserve University
Cleveland, Ohio

---

*Deceased

Victor Morgenroth Jr., BS, Pharmacy
Community Pharmacist
Ellicott City, Maryland

Charles E. Odegaard, PhD, Vice Chairman
Professor of Higher Education and President Emeritus
University of Washington
Seattle, Washington

Rozella M. Schlotfeldt, PhD
Professor of Nursing
Frances Payne Bolton School of Nursing
Case Western Reserve University
Cleveland, Ohio

William E. Smith Jr., PharmD
Director, Pharmacy and Central Services
Memorial Hospital Medical Center
Long Beach, California
and Associate Clinical Professor
School of Pharmacy
University of Southern California

Robert Straus, PhD
Professor and Chairman
Department of Behavioral Science
College of Medicine
University of Kentucky
Lexington, Kentucky

Lucy H. Joutz, Secretary

AACP ADVISORY COMMITTEE
FOR THE STUDY COMMISSION ON PHARMACY

Charles W. Bliven, DSc
Executive Secretary-Treasurer Emeritus
American Association of Colleges of Pharmacy
Bethesda, Maryland

Jere E. Goyan, PhD
Dean, School of Pharmacy
University of California
San Francisco, California

William J. Kinnard Jr., PhD
Dean, School of Pharmacy and Acting Dean of Graduate School
University of Maryland
Baltimore, Maryland

Arthur E. Schwarting, PhD, Chairman
Dean, School of Pharmacy
The University of Connecticut
Storrs, Connecticut

Lawrence C. Weaver, PhD, Ex officio
Dean, College of Pharmacy
University of Minnesota
Minneapolis, Minnesota

PREFACE

Pharmacy has not been oblivious to the criticism and questioning of the health service system which has been so evident in the United States during the past ten or fifteen years. There has been criticism of drug-related services from both without and within the profession of pharmacy. A number of leaders of pharmacy education have urged the necessity of an external examination of the state of the practice and education of pharmacists recognizing the vast changes which have occurred in biomedical knowledge and the expectations and demands of the public.

Responding to the recommendation and challenge laid down by its president, Dr. Arthur E. Schwarting, in an address in 1971, the American Association of Colleges of Pharmacy took prompt steps to consider and to implement a careful and external examination. An ad hoc committee consisting of Drs. Schwarting, John A. Biles, Jere E. Goyan, George P. Hager, William J. Kinnard Jr., and Charles W. Bliven, ex officio, was established. The committee consulted a number of educational leaders, prominent members of the pharmacy profession, and foundation officers. On the basis of the advice received, it was decided to ask that an independent body be commissioned, and I was invited to form and to chair it.

Eleven distinguished citizens were invited to serve as members. They represent diverse educational and professional backgrounds, but are united by a deep concern for the public good as it is enhanced through the services of the health professions. The Study Commission on Pharmacy has devoted more than two years to the examination of the practice of pharmacy as an integral part of the health service system and of the process of pharmacy education. It has conducted its study as a "group learning" exercise. No elaborate staff has been developed; rather, the Commission has operated as a "committee-of-the-whole" hearing all testimony, debating all issues, and joining unanimously in its findings.

The Study Commission has been greatly assisted by the views, advice, and counsel of eighty consultants whose names appear in the appendix at the end of this volume. The consultants have come from all facets of pharmacy and pharmacy education, from medicine and nursing, from hospitals and other health service organizations, from several levels of government, and from the pharmaceutical industry. The Commission expresses its thanks to all of these men and women who have given so generously of their time, experience, and interest.

The Commission is grateful for the generous financial support of its work furnished by the grants of The American Foundation for Pharmaceutical Education, The W. K. Kellogg Foundation, The Commonwealth Fund, The Edna McConnell Clark Foundation, and The Robert Wood Johnson Foundation.

Our thanks are also given to Mrs. Lucy Joutz of the AACP staff who has served skillfully as secretary of the Commission, and to Mr. Ernest Busch, our stenotypist.

The Study Commission on Pharmacy presents its Report to the American Association of Colleges of Pharmacy, to the profession, to the universities and colleges, to the health professions, and to all concerned members of the public. It is our hope that our efforts to appreciate the complexities of the present scene, to understand what the future may bring, and to suggest rational actions will be of substantial benefit to pharmacy through improved education of its members, and finally to the people of the United States as their health and well-being are enhanced by better drug-related services.

John S. Millis, Chairman
Cleveland, Ohio
September 1975

I. INTRODUCTION

The people of the United States are deeply concerned about drugs. All elements of our society are involved: health professionals, governmental officers, legislators, educators, pharmaceutical manufacturers, and consumers. There are many concerns about drugs: their purity, efficacy, and safety, their misuse by many individuals, their abuse by some—particularly by young people—their control, their costs, and their benefits.

Physicians, nurses, pharmacists, pharmaceutical manufacturers, and government officials are directly occupied with questions of drug efficacy and drug safety. Studies have reported data on the number of adverse reactions experienced by patients and the incidence of drug-induced disease. Cluff, Caranasos, and Stewart have stated:

> Intensive epidemiologic surveillance of hospitalized patients in the United States and abroad has shown that 2 to 5 percent of patient admissions to the medical and pediatric services of general hospitals are attributable to drug-induced disease. Five to 30 percent of patients experience adverse reactions to drugs during hospitalization. An unknown proportion of fetal abnormalities may be attributable to drugs taken by the mother during pregnancy or administered during parturition. An undetermined number of illnesses caused by drugs are responsible for visits of patients to physicians' offices. Conceivably, some diseases for which causes have not been demonstrated or which are widespread may have been induced by drugs.[1]

This identifies a great cost in human suffering and hundreds of millions of dollars annually in hospital and physicians' bills.

Pharmacists are naturally concerned. They are deeply involved with all the aspects of drugs that are discussed by physicians, government officers, and consumers. But also they are questioning their profession, their services, their roles, their economic welfare, and their future. The profession of pharmacy has undergone a revolution in the twentieth century. Some observers argue that pharmacy is now an obsolete or, at least, an obsolescent profession. Other observers describe pharmacy as a peripheral profession but point to gaps in health services involving drugs and urge that pharmacists undertake new duties to fill them.

To some observers, including the members of the Study Commission, the greatest concern regarding the nature of pharmacy arises from the unique circumstances which prevail in the pharmaceutical area. The unique circumstances relate to the discontinuities which exist between the generation of knowledge about drugs and the application of that knowledge in the clinical use of drugs. In nearly all other parts of the health care system there exists a functional interrelationship among the components involved in the education of health professionals, the delivery of health services to patients, and the search for new knowledge. Much of the responsibility for operating this interrelated system lies in the private sector. It is financed by philanthropy, government grants, and patient fees. It involves a corps of basic and clinical scientists seeking new knowledge and its application both to the delivery of health services to patients and to the education of health professionals. This interrelationship facilitates the broad and ready application of new knowledge and consequently is beneficial to the education of health professionals and to the delivery of health services.

In contrast, important parts of pharmacy—particularly the search for new knowledge—lie outside this framework. Most new knowledge is developed in the research laboratories of the pharmaceutical manufacturers. That knowledge is translated into new or improved drug products by the manufacturers and made available to prescribing physicians and dispensing pharmacists. Pharmaceutical manufacturing is a business enterprise. It exists solely upon the profits from the sale of its products. It receives no government grants or philanthropic gifts. The result is a drug armamentarium which is complex and of huge proportions. Many thousands of drug products are available. They are sold in a wide variety of dosage forms under generic names, trade names, and in combination with other drugs. The nature and practices of the pharmaceutical industry which lead to discontinuities among the components of research, education, and health service constitute a strong force in determining the form and nature of pharmacy.

Government regulation constitutes a second strong force in pharmacy. By law only those drugs considered pure, safe, and efficacious are allowed on the market. But government does not nor, in a free society, should it instruct a physician which, from a vast array of approved drugs, he should prescribe for his patients. It would seem that a third force is required and that it should be *professional* and *independent* of both government and industry.

Busy physicians prescribing for their patients are faced with a choice among many alternatives. The basic reference system which is available to them is a creation of the drug industry. Their journals are filled with drug advertising and they are visited by detail men whose essential job is to promote the use of their companies' products. Further, government and consumer groups are demanding that the physician consider drug costs also in making his decisions about drug therapy for his patients. Most physicians admit their need for professional assistance in making decisions of all kinds about drugs, but only a few believe that, at the present time, the assistance they require can be obtained from pharmacists. Perhaps the basic concern, therefore, is whether the profession of pharmacy can develop into a strong and effective third force to the end that optimal drug services will be acceptable to physicians and available to patients who require them.

It is against this background of deep and widespread concern about drugs, about pharmacy, and about pharmacists that the Study Commission on Pharmacy undertook its assignment to examine pharmacy education and to make recommendations designed to improve the education and training of pharmacists to the end that some of the drug-related problems may be solved and thereby the citizens of the nation may be better served. The Study Commission has based its examination and discussions upon three beliefs or presuppositions concerning drugs, pharmacy and pharmacists, and the education and training of professionals. The reader of this report should have these in mind as he follows its discussion and examines its conclusions.

1. The members of the Study Commission believe that in the absolute sense there is no completely safe nor universally effective drug. By definition a drug is a chemical used for diagnostic, therapeutic, or prophylactic purposes which produces chemical and biological effects in the body. In some individuals, under some conditions, in some combinations of circumstances of illness, diet, or time, drugs may produce unexpected and undesirable results or may prove therapeutically ineffective. Hence, any decision on drug therapy and its execution must involve a careful weighing of the expected benefits against the possible risks. Each decision requires a judgment. In the interest of the patient that judgment should be as highly informed as is humanly possible.

2. The members of the Study Commission believe that pharmacy should be an integral part, a subsystem, of what should be the health service delivery system of the nation. All pharmacists in their many roles practice within the health care system. Some of them are involved in the decision-making process concerning the utilization of drugs. All dispensing pharmacists are deeply involved in the execution of physicians' drug decisions. The pharmacists should have access to pertinent information about drugs and about their use by patients and participate in the weighing of expected benefits against possible risks and hence their professional judgment is of importance.

3. The character and quality of any professional service, whether it be that of a physician, an attorney, an engineer, or a pharmacist, is determined largely by the character, the quality, and the usefulness or practicality of the education and training he has received. There are many examples which one can cite where *wise and forceful action to improve education has resulted directly in higher standards of practice with clearly increased benefits to those who receive professional ser-*

vices. The ultimate objective of any professional education is to produce practitioners with knowledge, skill, and the motivation to provide an important, needed, and useful service. Any rational judgment about pharmacy education and any rational suggestion for change must be based upon a clear determination of the important, needed, and useful drug-related services which pharmacists can, do, and should provide.

The Study Commission began its consideration with the conceptualization of the health service delivery system as a matrix. The pharmacist is one of the elements of the matrix as he provides a drug-related service to a patient to facilitate the achievement of the ultimate aim of the system, namely the recovery or the maintenance of the health of that individual. Other elements of the matrix are: health professions—physicians, nurses, dentists, allied health professionals; the pharmaceutical industry; government agencies—at both the state and federal levels; health service institutions—hospitals, clinics, HMOs, nursing homes; educational institutions; health insurance organizations of diverse kinds; consumer groups. In this matrix there are interfaces between the pharmacist and each of the other individuals, institutions, and organizations. The Commission has proceeded to examine systematically many of these interfaces by consulting with appropriate representatives of the other elements of the matrix.

It is our hope that by this process we have gained knowledge and an appreciation of pharmacy and of pharmacists, an understanding of the forces which have and are producing change in pharmacy and in health care, and therefore the ability to forecast with some reliability the future course of change within the system and within pharmacy.

The ability to forecast for the future with some confidence is of paramount importance. Students beginning preparation for pharmacy in the fall of 1976 will not graduate until 1981 or 1982. They will not become experienced practitioners for another five or ten years. They will not be in leadership positions before 1995. Thus, students of 1976-81 must be educated for the practice of 1990-2020. The question which the Study Commission has attempted to answer is: What is the appropriate education for pharmacy practice in 1980, 1990, or 2000?

In the following eight chapters the Study Commission presents its understanding of the nature and the role of pharmacy, of the internal and external forces which produce continuing change, and of the functions and roles of pharmacists. In the final four chapters, the Commission sets forth its suggestions for changes in the educational system required in order adequately and appropriately to prepare the pharmacist of the future.

II. WHAT IS PHARMACY?

The most frequently encountered dictionary definition of pharmacy is "The art and science of compounding and dispensing drugs or medicines." Similarly, many dictionaries define the pharmacist as "One who compounds and dispenses drugs or medicines." Thus it is implied that the two concepts, "pharmacy" and "pharmacist," are congruent; that is, one can be derived from the other. One could define pharmacy and then state that the pharmacist is one who "does or practices" pharmacy. Conversely, one could define the pharmacist and then state that pharmacy is "what a pharmacist does."

Certainly the two concepts were congruent a century ago but they are not so in 1975. Circumstances have changed so radically that the two concepts must be approached independently. Thus, we shall attempt to define pharmacy as it is today and then attempt to describe in some detail in the following chapter those who are identified as pharmacists and to produce an acceptable definition.

The changes which have altered the relationship of pharmacy and pharmacists are well-known. A century ago medicines were compounded by a pharmacist or an apothecary in his pharmacy and dispensed or sold directly to a patient either upon the order or prescription of a physician or in many cases upon the direct request of the patient. The pharmacist compounded the medicine from plant or animal matter or from naturally occurring chemical materials. As the demand for medicines increased, a certain amount of division of labor appeared. Some pharmacists became wholesale providers of materials to other pharmacists furnishing processed or semi-processed plant or animal materials in the form of powders, extracts, and solutions. At that time what had been a purely cottage industry began to exhibit the first trends toward industrialization.

The great change in pharmacy began near the end of the nineteenth century with the rise of synthetic chemistry. The pharmacist was no longer limited to naturally occurring substances but had at his command a rapidly growing number of man-made materials. Beyond this it became possible to create new materials having specific chemical properties and with high probability of having desired pharmacological actions. The design, development, and production of synthetic chemicals and the drugs derived from them required both knowledge and facilities which the self-employed pharmacist did not possess. The knowledge was chemical and not exclusively pharmacological. The facilities were those of an industrial organization—laboratories, manufacturing machinery, wholesale distribution, and large amounts of capital.

The result of this change rapidly removed most of the compounding of drugs from the pharmacy and placed it in an industrial enterprise. The inevitable result has been a clear and substantial, although not absolute, separation of compounding and dispensing into two distinct activities. Over the years, more and more of the activity of compounding has become the responsibility of the manufacturer. For a time the manufacturer prepared the materials which the pharmacist assembled to prepare the dosage of medicine specified by the physician's prescription. Soon, however, it became more economical for the manufacturer to assume the responsibility for dosage formulation and even for packaging of frequently required quantities. The result of these changes was undoubtedly a much greater efficiency and large reduction in cost. The economy of scale of the concentration of scarce scientific and technological manpower and the opportunity for automation were available to large manufacturing corporations. None of them was available to the dispensing pharmacist. The result was that the public obtained more powerful drugs of more standardized quality and probably at a lower production cost, but the self-employed pharmacist ceased for the most part to be a compounder of drugs and became primarily a dispenser.

In spite of the radical changes in pharmacy and in the work of the self-employed pharmacist, the classical definition of pharmacy is still valid. Pharmacy is still the compounding and dispensing of drugs. True, compounding must be seen as a series of steps in a process of "putting together" drugs which is the root meaning of "compounding" although in general usage it may have a narrower meaning. Likewise, dispensing must be seen also as a series of steps of "weighing out," the root meaning of "dispensing" although again it may have a narrower meaning. In this view the two parts of pharmacy would be described by the following series of steps:

1. Compounding
    a. Discovery or invention
    b. Formulation
    c. Safety
    d. Efficacy
    e. Manufacture
2. Dispensing
    a. Product distribution
    b. Prescription filling
    c. Delivery to patients
    d. Drug administration

There is one sense in which this definition or description of pharmacy is incomplete. In the case of prescription drugs the process of pharmacy does not take a drug from invention to utilization by a patient except with the participation of an individual who is not a part of a pharmacy; that individual is the prescribing physician. A drug gets to the shelf of the pharmacy but is not dispensed to the ultimate user except upon the order of a physician. Hence, one must realize that there are two important discontinuities in the process—one between the drug manufacturer and the dispensing pharmacist, the other between the process of pharmacy and the authorized prescriber. A third discontinuity frequently develops—that between the intended behavior and the actual behavior of the patient with respect to the usage of the drug.

Although the classical definition of pharmacy may be valid without much stretching of the meaning of words, the Study Commission has found it more helpful to use a concept which is descriptive of all health services. *Pharmacy is a health service.* The only justification for inventing, manufacturing, distributing, prescribing, or dispensing drugs is that they can and do have a beneficial effect upon people who are ill and that drugs can cure disease, control disease, prevent disease, or ameliorate the sufferings of the victims of disease. One can conceive any health service, medicine, nursing, dentistry, or pharmacy, as a *knowledge system.* It is a system which generates or integrates knowledge about man in sickness and in health, takes knowledge from other sciences and arts, criticizes and organizes that knowledge, translates knowledge into technology, uses some knowledge to create products, devices, and instruments, transmits the knowledge through the education of practitioners and dissemination to others, to the end that an individual known as a patient may benefit from the particular knowledge system and its consequent skills. The thread which holds research, education and practice together in a rational system is *knowledge.* It is the knowledge which is the essential element and the application of the knowledge to the restoration or maintenance of health that is the ultimate justification and the intrinsic value of the system.

Pharmacy is just as much a *knowledge system* as is medicine. It generates, tests, applies, transmits, and utilizes knowledge. It differs from medicine in one very significant way. A substantial share of the knowledge of pharmacy is translated into a product that is a drug. A much smaller portion of the knowledge of internal medicine appears as apparatus. A more substantial portion of the knowledge of radiology appears in X-ray machines, accelerators, and radioisotope scanners. In surgery a growing amount of knowledge is appearing in the heart-lung machine, hip replacement materials, pacemakers, plastic blood vessel shunts. A large proportion of the knowledge of anesthesiology appears in the development, production, and utilization of appropriate chemical materials. The point is that pharmacy as a knowledge system differs from other health services not in its basic purpose nor in its intrinsic nature, but only in the degree to which some of its knowledge appears as a product.

The Study Commission advances the concept that pharmacy should be defined basically as a system which renders a health service by concerning itself with knowledge about drugs and their effects upon men and animals. Pharmacy generates knowledge about drugs, acquires relevant knowledge from the biological, chemical, physical, and behavioral sciences; it tests, organizes, and applies that knowledge. Pharmacy translates a substantial portion of that knowledge into drug products and distributes them widely to those who require them. Pharmacy knowledge is disseminated to physicians, pharmacists, and other health professionals and to the general public to the end that drug knowledge and products may contribute to the health of individuals and the welfare of society. The knowledge system of pharmacy through its therapeutic use is a substantial and significant segment of health care in the United States.

III. WHO ARE THE PHARMACISTS?

In Chapter II it was pointed out that the word "pharmacist" could not be derived at the present time from the definition of "pharmacy." In this chapter we will attempt to approach a definition by describing the individuals who are engaged in some portion of pharmacy viewed as a knowledge system and of their several roles and activities as pharmacists.

In a simple and legal sense one can identify a pharmacist as one who has been licensed or registered by a board of pharmacy in one of the fifty-two states or jurisdictions. In preparation for a study by Christopher A. Rodowskas Jr. and W. Michael Dickson[2] each board of pharmacy asked each registrant in its jurisdiction to fill out a questionnaire providing information upon many matters. The reports from the several jurisdictions were then collated, duplicate registrations eliminated, and national totals compiled by the authors. We begin the discussion of "Who are the Pharmacists?" with a brief analysis of the report.

Rodowskas and Dickson found that there were approximately 140,000 registered pharmacists in the United States in 1973. Of these about 20,000 were retired, unemployed, or engaged in an occupation other than pharmacy. Usable data on 103,340 active registered pharmacists were obtained, representing an 86.43 percent sample. This group reports a somewhat varied educational background as can be seen from Table 1.

One must conclude that it is impossible to define the pharmacist by a statement of a common formal educational preparation.

A second way to categorize pharmacists is by the principal place of current pharmacy activities. In Table 2 the number and the percentages of active registered pharmacists are reported by place of activity.

It is noted that the largest number, totaling approximately three-quarters of all registered pharmacists, are working in community pharmacies, fifty percent in independent establishments, twenty-six percent in chain stores. A breakdown of these nearly 80,000 registered pharmacists as between owners, manager-employees, and staff-employees is given in Table 3.

It is seen that thirty-eight percent of community pharmacists are proprietors and sixty-two percent are employees. It may be assumed that most of those working in hospitals and nursing homes are salaried employees. Surely all of those in government and education and most of those in manufacturing are also employees and not independent entrepreneurs. Thus we can conclude that seventy-one percent of the active registered pharmacists of the country depend upon salaries for their support and twenty-nine percent receive their income as proprietors of a business enterprise.

While the Rodowskas and Dickson study is undoubtedly the most complete and accurate report that is available, one must examine it for possible omissions. The figures for community pharmacists and for hospital and nursing home pharmacists are certainly complete. All such pharmacists are engaged in dispensing drugs. The laws of the several states and jurisdictions require that pharmacists be registered in order to dispense prescription drugs. However, a pharmacist does not now have to be registered or licensed to teach pharmacy, to hold a pharmacy position in government, or to work in a pharmaceutical capacity for a drug manufacturer or distributor, or even in a drug information center. Hence, one may conclude that the figures may understate the number engaged in pharmacy activities other than those of community and hospital pharmacy. There is some evidence to substantiate this conjecture, particularly in industrial pharmacy. However, there are no reliable figures to reveal the total number of persons engaged in pharmacy activities including both those registered and unregistered.

The information in the Rodowskas and Dickson study provides an insight as to where pharmacists work and about the source from which they receive their livelihoods. It gives some clues to the question of what pharmacists do, but it is far from definitive. There have been several detailed studies of the activities of community and of hospital pharmacists, but none concerning those otherwise occupied. The Study Commission has reviewed many of the studies and has interviewed a large number of individuals whose testimony has given a reasonably clear picture, at least qualitatively, of the activities of pharmacists in their several work environments.

Independent Community Pharmacists

The activities of pharmacists in independent community pharmacies can be described only in terms of a broad spectrum. In the first place the pharmacies vary quite widely in their character and the nature of their activities. In the second place the responsibilities of the pharmacist vary in community pharmacies of the same type. At one end of the spectrum a few pharmacies confine themselves principally or even exclusively to the dispensing of prescription drugs and can be described as prescription pharmacies or apothecary shops. In such institutions the pharmacist is occupied nearly full time in purely pharmacy activities. He is engaged in the operations of pouring, counting, and labeling the materials called for by a physician's prescription. To support these activities he is responsible for the purchase, protection, and care of the drugs obtained from the manufacturer or wholesaler. In many cases the pharmacist uses assistants to perform some routine tasks while he supervises their work to insure the accuracy of the dispensing process. Freed from some of the routine tasks the pharmacist is able to devote more time to delivering services to the patient in addition to delivering the drug to him. Often he maintains a medication profile for each of his patients, recording all prescriptions, individual patient drug idiosyncrasies, and the purchase or usage of over-the-counter drugs. By reviewing the drug profile he is able to note the possibility of drug interactions and to call the attention of the prescribing physician to them. Further he is free to talk directly to patients receiving prescriptions to reinforce physician instructions and to clarify the details of the utilization and administration of the drugs acquired. Some pharmacies provide facilities for private patient counseling.

At the other end of the spectrum is the large and complex drugstore dealing in prescription drugs, over-the-counter medications, cosmetics, tobacco products, candy, liquor, greeting cards, magazines, and a wide variety of other products. In such a situation the staff pharmacist spends most of his time filling prescriptions and in the related tasks of maintaining the drug inventory and its safety. If the pharmacist is the proprietor of the store he is responsible for the management of a complex retail establishment and the tasks involved therein. Some such pharmacies do maintain patient drug records and do provide some patient counseling; however, such services are less frequently encountered than in the apothecary-type establishment. If the prescription filling activities do not require the full-time efforts of the pharmacist, particularly the staff-employee person, he may also function as a sales person, retailing the other goods offered.

Other pharmacies fall in between the two extremes of the spectrum described. The size of the operation, its location, its clientele, the size of the prescription business, and the personal motivation and preferences of the pharmacists involved all seem to determine the character of the operation.

Chain Community Pharmacies

The community pharmacies owned and operated by a chain do not vary so widely in character. Chain stores tend to be larger and more complex in their activities than independent pharmacies. The dispensing of prescribed drugs is frequently but a minor part of a large retailing operation. The pharmacist who is naturally a staff-employee concentrates upon filling prescriptions. In some operations he uses a variety of assistants to increase the number of prescriptions filled in a day, thereby reducing labor costs and permitting lower charges to patients. Some chain pharmacies do maintain patient drug profiles, but not with the regularity seen in the apothecary-type shops nor in a number of independent pharmacies. Those pharmacists who are appointed as managers devote their attention to the entire operation and spend comparatively little time upon activities directly connected with the pharmacy as such.

Hospital Pharmacies

Hospital pharmacies and the activities of pharmacists within them must also be described in terms of a spectrum for they are far from homogeneous in character. At one end is the hospital pharmacy which is nothing more than an apothecary shop which happens to be located in a hospital, usually in the basement. The pharmacist is engaged in providing the drugs ordered by staff physicians to be administered to their patients being treated in the hospital. The essential difference from community practice is that the pharmacist responds to a drug order of a physician rather than a prescription submitted by a patient. Rather than handing the drug to the patient it is delivered by messenger or pneumatic tube to a nurse who administers the ordered dosage to the patient.

At the other end of the spectrum is the hospital pharmacy which provides a complex and complete drug service to the patients, the physicians, and the nurses of the hospital. Drugs are furnished in response to physician orders but frequently by the unit dose system whereby the nursing staff is released from the necessity of counting out individual dosages and maintaining stocks of drugs in patient areas. In some hospital pharmacy systems the pharmacist is frequently seen participating directly in patient services. He may participate actively with the hospital's Pharmacy and Therapeutics Committee assisting in the development of the institution's drug formulary and in the solution of drug-related problems of the institution. He may be responsible for obtaining the drug history of admitted patients. He may make patient rounds with physicians and nurses thus being available for consultation on specific drug problems. He may be assigned responsibility for monitoring the drug regimen of a patient and the patient's reaction to the drug therapy. Interestingly, in many well-developed hospital pharmacy systems the pharmacist is devoting increasing attention to special types of compounding. The pharmacist is responsible for mixing intravenous solutions and sometimes for their administration to patients. A few pharmacists are engaged in the compounding of solutions containing radioactive materials used in programs of chemotherapy and various testing procedures.

Pharmacists engaged in activities closely related to hospitalized patients have come to describe themselves as "clinical pharmacists" for they are more directly and continuously engaged in the process of patient care. These pharmacists continue the historic role of dispensers of drugs but they have developed a variety of other services to assist in the safe and efficacious utilization of drugs by patients most of whom are seriously ill and are ministered to in a complex and technologically sophisticated institution.

Nursing Home Pharmacies

Once again pharmacy services and pharmacist activities in nursing homes must be described in terms of a spectrum. At one end is the nursing home, usually small, which purchases from a community pharmacy the prescriptions written for its patients by attending physicians. The activity of the pharmacist, except where written reviews of drug therapy for patients at regular intervals are required, is identical to that required in filling a prescription handed to him by a patient who appears at his store. The only difference is that the drug called for is delivered by messenger and not directly to the patient. The other end of the spectrum is represented in a large nursing home which develops on the premises a hospital-type pharmacy managed by a pharmacist. The activity of the pharmacist may vary from merely filling prescriptions to direct participation in patient care involving drug use monitoring and regular patient visitation and reporting to the appropriate visiting physician.

An interesting development has taken place in some situations. The nursing home contracts with a community pharmacist to provide the prescriptions required and also, for a fee, to give continuing advice and to monitor the drug usage of the patients involved. In such a situation the pharmacist visits the nursing home regularly, inspects the drug records of the patients, communicates with physicians concerning his observations, and counsels with patients and the nursing staff. Studies of some of these arrangements report that actual cost savings have resulted from regular monitoring of drug utilization and communication with prescribing physicians. Substantial reductions in drug use by patients have resulted and the consequent savings have more than offset the fees paid to the consulting pharmacist. There is now a group of young pharmacists who describe themselves as "drug consultants" and devote themselves exclusively to providing their services to nursing homes.

One must observe that the evidence indicates that many, if not most, nursing homes provide inadequate pharmacy services to their patients. Most nursing homes are small and cannot afford the full-time or even the part-time services of a well-trained pharmacist. There are few consultant pharmacists available and again the cost of their services discourages their use. Improvement in pharmacy services to nursing home patients has been demonstrated to be possible and practical. Recently promulgated federal regulations mandate many of these improved drug services if nursing homes are to qualify for reimbursement for services to Medicare and Medicaid patients.

Ambulatory Health Service Organizations and Institutions

A new field of pharmacy practice is developing in connection with the growth of ambulatory care facilities of many kinds. In outpatient clinics, in HMOs, in prepaid health care plans, and in group practice organizations more comprehensive and consistent pharmacy services are appearing. In these situations the activities of pharmacists differ in scope from those traditionally seen in the community pharmacy. As clinics have expanded in size and comprehensiveness it has been necessary to include services other than those rendered by physicians and nurses. Drug-related services are among the first to be included and pharmacists are found on the staffs of a variety of clinics. As would be expected, their responsibilities begin with the dispensing of drugs to patients as they are prescribed. However, one finds examples of other services being performed. Being on the premises furnishes many more opportunities for consultation concerning drugs and drug problems between pharmacists on the one hand and physicians and nurses on the other. The pharmacist in such situations also can maintain quite complete patient drug profiles. He is the representative of the institution at the point of the delivery of the prescribed drug to the patient. He has the opportunity to communicate with the patient and to instruct him as to administration of his medication. He has had opportunity to discuss the most appropriate information with the prescribing physician and others to insure consistency. In some cases the pharmacist plays a larger role as patient advisor. In the Group Health Cooperative of Puget Sound, pharmacists in a program approved by physicians conduct formal instruction sessions for patients on long-term drug therapy regimens such as are required for diabetes control, hypertension control, and anticoagulant therapy. In one large metropolitan hospital outpatient division pharmacists and nurses, under the supervision of a physician, conduct diabetes and hypertension ambulatory clinics, see the patients upon their regular visits, develop drug and patient records, observe patient compliance, and refer appropriate patients for consultation with a physician. One can cite a number of other examples where health professionals of several kinds including pharmacists are working collaboratively.

Pharmaceutical Manufacturing

There are no complete and reliable data on the activities, roles, and employment of pharmacists in the pharmaceutical industry. It is certain that nearly 5,000 registered pharmacists are so employed. However, we do not know how many individuals who have been initially educated as pharmacists, but have not continued their registration, are actively at work within the industry. It is clear from the testimony given to the Study Commission that there are individuals educated and sometimes registered as pharmacists holding positions at every step and in every subsystem of that portion of pharmacy designated as the pharmaceutical industry.

In the activities of research and development of new drug products there are pharmacists. Many of these individuals have taken graduate degrees in relevant scientific disciplines such as pharmacology, organic chemistry, biochemistry, physiology, or pharmaceutical chemistry. The same statement can be made about the involvement of pharmacists in the subsystem of clinical trials of new drugs.

There is ample evidence that pharmacists are heavily involved in the step of dosage formulation. Several consultants have stated that if pharmacists were not available to manufacturing firms for this responsibility, personnel would have to be trained and developed by the industry.

Pharmacists are involved in the manufacturing step and their work in quality control is mentioned frequently. Again, the phenomenon of additional training in a cognate discipline such as physical chemistry or chemical engineering is observed.

Pharmacists are involved in distribution of pharmaceutical products, in marketing, sales, and wholesale distribution. There are probably between 1,500 and 2,000 pharmacists employed as detail men carrying information concerning pharmaceutical products directly to physicians and to dispensing pharmacists. The practice of pharmaceutical manufacturers varies on this point. Some companies use pharmacists almost exclusively as detail men; others employ very few pharmacists. There is a change occurring which is worthy of note. In the past pharmaceutical manufacturers have concentrated heavily upon contacts with prescribing physicians as the decision makers concerning the use of their products. Currently many firms are seeking direct communication with dispensing pharmacists in recognition of their growing influence upon the choice of drug products to be used. The detail man is therefore calling on both physicians and pharmacists. This change must indicate that drug manufacturers now conceive the pharmacist as a more influential member of the drug distribution system than he has been in recent decades.

Pharmacists are employed in the preparation of written materials which manufacturers must provide to physicians, pharmacists, and regulatory bodies such as the FDA. In short, pharmacists can be found in the pharmaceutical manufacturing industry at every level and in every activity involved. However, they must function in a multidisciplinary environment with a host of others with different educational backgrounds and professional training, although within the team they retain a clear responsibility for dosage formulation.

Drug Information Centers

A number of drug information centers have been developed in the past decade. These are institutions designed to furnish information required principally by physicians to deal with drug-related problems and to improve drug prescribing. They also receive some requests for information from pharmacists and from nurses. Such centers are generally operated by pharmacists and frequently are associated with colleges of pharmacy. The pharmacists who operate them have quite generally added to their competence by acquiring knowledge and skill in information and communications theory and management.

In some large and well-developed hospital pharmacy systems, a drug information service is an integral part of the organization. Such services are available to provide information to the medical, nursing, and pharmacy staff and are quite heavily used. In a few instances such drug information centers make their services available to nearby hospitals and to community pharmacists of the region. In some cases drug information and poison control centers are joined into a single agency. However, the two types of information centers do not appear to be easily joined. This may be due to the fact that drug information centers are generally manned by pharmacists, while poison control centers are generally under the supervision of physicians operated under governmental standards, and are viewed as a part of the community apparatus to respond to medical emergencies.

After this rapid review of where pharmacists are working, and what they are doing, we return to the question: "What is a pharmacist?" It is abundantly clear that pharmacists practice in *one of the steps of a system* or in *one of the subsystems of a process* which we identify as "pharmacy." Thus, it is impossible to refer to *the pharmacist;* rather, we must speak in the plural of *the pharmacists* since their activities cover a spectrum and no single individual is engaged in all the activities encompassed in that spectrum. True, two-thirds of the pharmacists of the United States are engaged in the dispensing of drugs in community pharmacies and an additional eleven or twelve percent are engaged substantially in the dispensing of drugs in hospitals and other institutions furnishing medical services. Still there are pharmacists engaged in every other pharmaceutical activity one can name. Thus, one must define a pharmacist as an individual who is engaged in *one of the steps of a process called pharmacy.* We cannot define a pharmacist as one who practices pharmacy. Rather, he must be defined as one who practices a part of pharmacy which is determined by the activities carried on in one of the subsystems of the total system of pharmacy.

Within most of the steps or subsystems the pharmacist shares responsibility with many people with different educational and professional backgrounds—scientists, physicians, engineers, managers, marketers, hospital administrators, and many others. In only one of the subsystems, that of dispensing prescription drugs, does the pharmacist maintain dominance and control, and then only under the orders of a physician.

There is an observation to be made concerning the knowledge and skills of pharmacists. As they find their individual roles within one step of the process they all have a common body of knowledge about drugs. However, to fulfill their particular roles they add to this common core knowledge and skill taken from another science, technology, or discipline. The research pharmacist has added chemistry, physiology, or pharmacology; the manufacturing pharmacist has added chemical engineering or physical chemistry; the distributive pharmacist has added marketing and sales; the community pharmacist has added management and retail selling; the hospital pharmacist has added systems management and health care administration; the drug information pharmacist has added information theory and technology. Thus, one must describe the pharmacist as a bivalent or polyvalent person. It is the *common* denominator of drug knowledge *and* the *differentiated additional knowledge and skill* required by his particular role which characterize and describe him.

The thoughts just expressed immediately raise the question of whether the pharmacists have become specialists. Pharmacists are differentiated by what they know, what they can do, and how and where they practice. However, such differentiation is unlike the differentiation in medicine which we call specialization. The medical specialist who knows more about a particular disease, organ, or organ system than does any other kind of physician or any other professional is monovalent. The differentiated pharmacist probably knows little more about pharmacy as such than do most other pharmacists and he possesses no more than many other kinds of professionals of the knowledge which he has acquired from other fields and disciplines, but he is bivalent.

TABLE 1. Active Registered Pharmacists by Years of Undergraduate Education

	Number	Percent
1. Less than 4 years	11,796	11.4
2. Four years	54,900	53.1
3. Five years	28,820	27.9
4. Six years	2,268	2.2
5. No degree received	4,200	4.1
6. Not reported	1,356	1.3
	103,340	100.0

TABLE 2. Active Registered Pharmacists by Principal Place of Pharmacy Practice

	Number	Percent
1. Community pharmacy-independent	52,007	50.3
2. Community pharmacy-chain	27,145	26.3
3. Hospitals and nursing homes	14,859	14.4
4. Manufacturing and distribution	4,838	4.7

TABLE 2 *(continued)*

	Number	Percent
5. Government, teaching, and other pharmaceutical capacities	3,136	3.0
6. Not reported	1,355	1.3
	103,340	100.0

TABLE 3. Community Pharmacists by Employment Status

	Number	Percent
1. Sole owner	18,633	23.5
2. Partner	11,448	14.5
3. Manager-employee	13,921	17.6
4. Assistant manager-employee	7,454	9.4
5. Staff-employee	26,228	33.2
6. Other	968	1.2
7. Not reported	500	0.6
	79,152	100.0

IV. PHARMACY AND THE PUBLIC INTEREST

The very word "pharmacy" has had an ominous tone throughout history. The word is derived from the Greek "pharmakon" meaning a "poison." Thus, it is natural that society has long been concerned about drugs and their utilization, realizing that just as they may possess powers to heal and cure they also can and do pose threats to life and health of those who consume them. It should be no surprise therefore that pharmacy and those engaged therein should be subject to a substantial societal control through laws, licensure, and regulation by organized governments at many levels. Such control and regulation have had and will continue to have great effect upon the development of pharmacy and upon the practice of pharmacists. Thus, an examination of pharmacy and the public interest is highly germane to the consideration of the future of pharmacy and the education of its future practitioners.

In the United States the public interest concerning drugs has been expressed at both federal and state levels. The federal legislation has been based upon the regulation of interstate commerce and therefore has been concerned primarily with pharmaceutical products—their quality, safety, and efficacy. The state legislation has been based upon the responsibility to protect the safety and welfare of the citizens of the jurisdiction and has been concerned with the qualifications of those who prescribe and dispense drugs, the places where drugs may be safely maintained and dispensed, and products involved in intrastate commerce.

The earliest federal drug legislation was in response to the need to assure purity, uniformity, and stability. Standards of quality were established for drug products sold in interstate commerce. A federal bureau, the Food and Drug Administration (FDA), was created to set standards and regulations and to monitor the quality of drugs. As new drugs became more powerful in their beneficial effect they also became more hazardous. The next concern of the federal government, therefore, was for drug safety. Legislation placed responsibility upon the FDA for regulation of the manufacture and distribution of drugs with reference to their safety to the consumer. Other legislation established a special category of "controlled drugs" and initially placed responsibility for control of such substances upon a division of the Treasury Department but it is now assigned to the Drug Enforcement Agency of the Justice Department. Regulations resulted to require particular handling, procedures, and records on the part of both physicians and pharmacists. Most recently legislation has been enacted to ensure the efficacy of drugs offered on the market. Again, the FDA has been given responsibility and substantial authority for this aspect of pharmacy.

In discharging its several responsibilities the FDA has found it appropriate to establish two categories of drugs—those which may be dispensed only upon prescription and those which can be sold without prescription and which are usually referred to as over-the-counter (OTC) drugs. The discrimination between these two categories of drug products is made not upon the basis of differences in quality, safety, or efficacy, but allegedly upon the basis of the risks associated with their use and the ease or difficulty of transmitting information about the drug to the ultimate user. Thus, an OTC product is presumably one whose label can carry sufficient information to the purchaser to ensure that it may be used with safety and benefit if taken in accordance with the instructions of the label. A prescription drug is one with which there is a risk associated or for which such a satisfactory label cannot be prepared. Thus, the FDA has become concerned with drug information since the basic classifications of drug products depend upon the adequacy, simplicity, and completeness of knowledge about each drug. With respect to prescription drugs the FDA requires a package insert addressed to the prescribing physician carrying information about chemical and pharmaceutical qualities, efficacy, hazards, and indicated usage. Recently the Agency has required, for some drugs, that package inserts be delivered to the patient in order to provide the ultimate user with additional information concerning the drug, its usage, and its effects. Another federal concern is with the accuracy of claims made in advertising the efficacy of OTC drugs.

Most recently the federal government has become concerned with another aspect of pharmacy—that is the cost of drugs. With the enactment of Medicare and Medicaid legislation, the cost of medical care for millions of American citizens has been assumed by the federal government. As the costs of such care have risen, more and more attention has been paid to the prices of prescription drugs, and regulations are now being proposed to control the charges which can be made. Thus, it can be said that the federal government is involved in setting standards, monitoring, and regulating almost every aspect of pharmacy, and thereby affecting the practice of those involved in the system.

The concern of the several states was initially and still is principally with the determination of standards of competency of the individuals involved in prescribing and dispensing drugs, i.e., physicians and pharmacists. Quite early in our history the several states decided that in order to protect the well-being of their citizens it was necessary to license practitioners of medicine and pharmacy. State boards of medicine and of pharmacy were created to set standards of education and competence and to certify the competence of the physician and pharmacist through licensure. As public concern arose over quality, safety, and efficacy of drugs, it was necessary for the states to join with the federal government to regulate both intrastate and interstate distribution and sale of drug products.

There are other concerns of state governments, such as the safety and adequacy of the places of business in which drugs are dispensed, the control of dangerous drugs and poisons, and the enforcement of drug abuse laws. Most recently a number of states have added further regulations concerning the practice of pharmacists requiring the maintenance of patient drug records, and the state of Washington requires that pharmacists provide information as to the use of the drug directly to patients at the time of dispensing a drug. The states of Florida, Kansas, Ohio, New Jersey, Indiana, and California have legislated requirements designed to encourage continued competence of pharmacists by mandating continuing education for the pharmacist to maintain his registration. The states of Nevada, Colorado, Washington, Minnesota, and Oklahoma have enacted similar laws which will become effective in the next few years.

From this recital it is clear that pharmacy and pharmacists are among the most regulated and controlled segments of our society. Pharmacy is much more regulated and controlled than medicine, nursing, or dentistry. The pharmaceutical industry is more regulated and controlled than most manufacturers. One may well ask why this is so. In just what way is the public interest so special that it must be protected by such complete regulation in a society which claims to place freedom as its highest value? There is one way in which pharmacy differs from other health services which may explain in part the special way in which we view pharmacy; that difference lies in the feasibility or existence of voluntary control and regulation.

Recent years have seen the development of new and highly sophisticated surgical procedures such as open heart surgery and kidney transplants. Such procedures have the potential of saving and extending the lives of desperately ill patients. By their very nature, however, such procedures are hazardous and their potential for harm is great. Yet society has not found it necessary to enact legislation to control the utilization of the newly developed techniques. One reason is that there has developed a substantial voluntary system upon which reliance is placed to protect the public interest. Beyond basic licensure, physicians are examined and certified by voluntary but prestigious national boards for special knowledge, skill, and competence. Furthermore, complex surgery cannot be performed outside of a hospital and hospitals are accredited by a voluntary agency and frequently licensed by the state. A surgeon cannot operate in a hospital without being granted staff privileges which are dependent upon review by his peers and their acceptance of his competence.

The situation in pharmacy is quite different. The increase in the power of a new drug may be just as great or greater than that of a newly devised surgical procedure. The potential for benefit of the newly developed drug is great, but so is its potential for harm. However, unlike surgery, there is no voluntary system which selects those who are specially competent to prescribe it, nor the institutions in which it is to be administered. Every licensed physician, dentist, osteopath is free to prescribe any and all approved drugs. Other health professionals, e.g., the podiatrist, are free to prescribe drugs utilized in their area of practice responsibility. In surgery the system operates to permit the usage of the most dangerous procedures only by an ever more rigorously limited group of practitioners. Just the reverse happens in pharmacy. Drugs are prescribed and administered by an increasingly broad spectrum of health professionals. The usage of antibiotics by dentists is increasing more rapidly than by any medical specialty. Within but a few years psychiatrists have become constant prescribers of the newly developed and very powerful psychotropic drugs. It can be well argued that in the absence of a reliable system of voluntary control, it is necessary that in pharmacy there be an ever growing set of controls fashioned by legislation and enforced by governmental bureaus. Further, legal control is much more easily applied to the manufacture and distribution of a product than it is to the individual health professional.

Few people will argue that it is unnecessary for society to exercise a substantial amount of control and regulation over pharmacy in order to protect the public interest and the life and health of citizens. However, there are a number of well-informed and highly competent people who feel that the degree of control imposed by government is so excessive that the public interest is poorly served in a number of ways. There are others who admit that governmental control is not always consistent but that while some segments are overcontrolled, other segments are not controlled enough. It is true that the requirements of the FDA which must be met by a pharmaceutical manufacturer as to quality, safety, and efficacy involve more testing and more voluminous reports than are demanded in any other industrial country. It costs more money and takes more time to get a new drug cleared for marketing in the United States than in England or in a number of European countries. British physicians are able to use new drugs which are not permitted on the market in the United States and are not available to American physicians and their patients. Further, the high cost of carrying a new drug through development, testing, and clearance by the FDA has resulted in some decrease in the number of new drugs introduced. Obviously as the cost of introducing a drug rises, the number produced will decline.

There are arguments being raised against the proposed federal government plan to insist upon generic prescribing by limiting reimbursement to the minimum available price of each specific drug compound in its chemically equivalent form. Many physicians and scientists argue that not all chemically equivalent drugs are biologically and therefore therapeutically equivalent. Consumer advocates feel that the control of drug advertising is inadequate and not properly protective of the public interest. Other critics stress that no drug is absolutely safe and that the test of an understandable label is no guarantee that an over-the-counter drug is sufficiently safe in the hands of uninformed or misinformed laymen.

Ironically, despite the significant amount and force of existing controls on the manufacture and distribution of drugs, there is evidence that most drugs are frequently inappropriately used by patients. Inappropriate use involves taking too little or too much of a prescribed medication or mixing medications in ways that produce adverse effects, or self-medicating with drugs leftover from previous prescriptions, or self-medicating with over-the-counter remedies that have no therapeutic effect for the symptoms for which they are used. These and other examples of the misuse of drugs result in a significant though unmeasurable waste of money and produce frequent problems of drug ineffectiveness, toxicity, or adverse interaction. These kinds of problems do not appear to be responsive to governmental controls. They require a better system of distribution of knowledge about drugs, a topic that is discussed in Chapter VI.

It is clear that the question of governmental control of pharmacy is still being debated and requires continued consideration and that there will be changes in the years to come. The ratio of possible risk to possible benefit is difficult, if not impossible, to determine prospectively with accuracy. Until we have much more knowledge about many drugs and their effect upon the human body we will continue to debate how best to protect the public interest and at the same time to encourage the advancement of knowledge and the progress of medical science.

A substantial amount of time has been devoted to this discussion of pharmacy and the public interest. We have done so because governmental control and regulation is probably the strongest external force shaping and determining the evolution of pharmacy, and thereby the practice of pharmacists. There is no reason to expect that the future will bring any appreciable decrease in such control; in fact, the reverse is more likely. As new and more powerful drugs are developed even greater regulation may be deemed necessary. Thus, in considering the future of pharmacy and pharmacists we must recognize the continuing strong influence of society's concern for the public interest.

V. ECONOMICS AND THE PHARMACIST

If governmental control and regulation have been the strongest external forces acting upon the development of pharmacy and the practice of pharmacists, economic forces have been a close second. Economics almost alone has been responsible for the separation between the compounding and dispensing functions of pharmacy. As the science of synthetic chemistry developed, the source of drugs was expanded rapidly and very greatly. The materials from which drugs were compounded had to be manufactured rather than extracted from naturally available materials. Such manufacturing was economic only when it involved large quantities and a concentration of capital and facilities. The pharmacist could not compete with the much more efficient commercial manufacturer. A second economy was realized by combining the manufacturing of the raw material and the production of the finished drug dosage. Again this involved economies of scale and the availability of capital and facilities. A third economy appeared as drug research and development began. These activities required the efforts of highly trained and highly competent scientists. The costs of such personnel can be borne only in the well-managed and adequately financed research organizations. The cost of increasing requirements for quality, safety, and efficacy imposed by government are great and again can be met only by an industrial organization with a large output and large sales. In short, no cottage industry, whether it be textile weaving or drug compounding, can compete economically with a well-developed industrial enterprise furnishing the same product. Thus, economic forces changed the self-employed pharmacist from a compounder and dispenser of drugs into primarily a dispenser.

A second economic force acting upon the pharmacist arises out of the long-established custom of providing compensation of the pharmacist in the retail price of the dispensed drug. This arrangement provided no problem to the pharmacist a century ago when he was both the compounder and the dispenser of the drug requested by a patient. The patient viewed the fee which he paid as covering the materials used, but also the knowledge and the skill of the pharmacist required to compound the drug and dispense it with proper regard for the safety and welfare of the buyer. The special knowledge and skill of the pharmacist were very evident and probably willingly paid for. As compounding became manufacturing and the self-employed pharmacist became primarily a dispenser, the special knowledge and skill became less evident. The patient viewed dispensing as a comparatively simple merchandising task meriting no greater markup over the wholesale cost than is customary in a retail transaction. The pharmacist was trapped into depending for his livelihood upon what he could add as a markup on a product, competition largely determining the markup on drug products sold at retail.

The self-employed pharmacist, in order to survive economically, had but three choices. First, he could diversify and increase the number of other products to be sold at retail—cosmetics, home remedies, tobacco, liquor, candy, magazines, electrical appliances, and garden tools. As a retailer of a broad line of goods he could survive economically, but at the cost of spending less and less time in activities identified as those of a professional pharmacist involved in a direct health service to patients. Second, he could join with other pharmacists and with managers, financial experts, and other retail merchandisers to form a chain store corporation. This step would provide economy of scale, quantity purchasing with greater wholesale and retail discounts, more expert management and more adequate financing. Third, he could seek an especially favorable location such as a physicians' office building where the number of prescriptions presented would be of sufficient magnitude to occupy him full time and where he could concentrate more of his time upon the sale of pharmaceuticals. Thus, economic considerations have dictated to a large degree how and where a great number, in fact the majority, of pharmacists practice.

The traditional practice of providing for the compensation of the dispensing pharmacist by a markup in the price of the prescribed product provided to the patient has determined the concept of the dispensing act held both by the pharmacist and by the patient. It has been viewed as being the provision of a product. It has generally not been viewed as the provision of a health service to a patient. The system or process of pharmacy is designed to transfer knowledge, a part of which is contained in a drug product, to the ultimate benefit for the patient for whom that product has been prescribed. The process of dispensing does deliver the product; but it may very easily fail to include delivering the information and knowledge to the patient which may be required for the most effective utilization of the drug. The patient does not expect nor request that information. The pharmacist is not compensated for the delivery of knowledge and has no economic incentive to provide it. One can imagine a situation in which a pharmacist discovers from the patient drug record that the prescription presented is identical to that given to the patient by another physician a few days before. If the pharmacist calls the second physician to report the duplicate prescription, it is at the expense of the opportunity to sell the second prescription. Or if a pharmacist notices that a patient to whom he is delivering a prescription is purchasing an over-the-counter drug which will likely produce an adverse reaction when taken in conjunction with the prescription, he undoubtedly should advise the patient not to make the purchase. However, such advice is given at the expense of a prospective sale and profit to the pharmacist. Not only is there no economic incentive to communicate with the patient, there is the reverse incentive *not* to communicate.

In recent years a new economic force has arisen which has a strong effect upon the practice of the pharmacist; that is the rapid spread of health insurance plans that include full or partial reimbursement for the costs of prescription drugs. There are such provisions in Medicaid, in a number of union health insurance plans, in several medical foundation programs, and in the program for prepaid prescriptions organized by retail pharmacists in several areas of the country. As would be expected, the introduction of third-party payers has been a strong influence upon the economics of retail pharmacy and the compensation of pharmacists. All insurance plans must strive to control the costs of the benefits they provide. Thus, there is a strong tendency to set maximum allowable prices. Since the costs of drug products to the retail pharmacist vary with his source of supply and particularly with the volume of his purchases, the pharmacist, who must buy at a disadvantage but cannot charge more than a set maximum, receives less for his dispensing services than some of his competitors.

The practice of the retail pharmacist has been affected by this force of economic change. A number of innovations have appeared. First, some pharmacists have agreed with third-party payers on a dispensing fee. Instead of applying a standard percentage markup to the acquisition cost, he receives his cost plus a flat fee for each prescription. In such a plan the pharmacist's services become clearly visible and therefore can be defined and specified. Thus, patient drug records can be called for, instruction to patients can be specified, and the pharmacist can be directly compensated for services actually rendered. The idea of a dispensing fee first employed in Medicaid regulations appears to be spreading. It appears in a number of the agreements between nursing homes and the retail pharmacists who fill prescriptions for the patients of the institution. However, it should be noted that problems have been encountered in establishing a prescription fee system. The bargaining power in setting the amounts of the fee is heavily weighted against the individual pharmacist in dealing with a government bureau or a large insurance company. Further, the system can be abused in ordering inappropriately frequent refills. Still the dispensing fee system has much to recommend it and with proper surveillance and good faith can be expected to work well.

A second change in the practice of the retail pharmacist appears as an accommodation to the increase in record keeping necessary for reimbursement by a third-party payer. As more and more of the prescriptions provided by a pharmacist are paid by someone other than the patient, the pharmacist must devote substantial time and attention to financial records, to filling out forms, and seeking reimbursement; this naturally involves added costs. Some pharmacists have found that the only way to meet these costs is through the increased utilization of the advanced technology of the computer. Not only does this make the cost of added paperwork bearable, but it also gives the opportunity for much greater efficiency in other aspects of operating a retail pharmacy including inventory control, ordering, patient records, and drug utilization data.

A third change is the appearance of retail pharmacy cooperatives. In a few regions pharmacists have joined together for purchasing at wholesale or directly from manufacturers. This gives the independent pharmacist the means to obtain his drugs at the price which is available to a chain operation or to a large hospital. Thus, a degree of organization and institutionalization is beginning to appear in independent retail pharmacy.

There is one sociopolitical fact that has had a large economic impact on pharmacy; that is the public policy concerning the support of research and development in pharmacy. In general, the search for knowledge and new technology in the area of the health services has been historically, and continues to be viewed, as so clearly in the public interest that it is largely supported by philanthropic and public funds. Research in the biomedical sciences, in the clinical branches of medicine, in nursing, and in dentistry is paid for almost exclusively by foundations, philanthropies, universities, and agencies of the federal government such as the National Institutes of Health and the National Science Foundation. In sharp contrast most of the research and development in pharmacy is paid out of the profits of pharmaceutical manufacturing.

It is of interest to note the differences in public policy with regard to tax support of industrial research and development. If one ranks the industries of the country in order of public support of their research and development efforts, one finds that pharmacy ranks at the bottom of the list. Sixty to seventy-five percent of the costs of research and development in such areas as transportation and electronics are paid for by tax funds. In machine tools, foods, instruments, and heavy chemicals, the federal contribution accounts for a quarter or a third of the costs of research. In the drug industry less than three percent of research and development costs come from tax sources.[3] It is fair to say that pharmacy research and development is at this time not a public business, but rather a private business dependent almost exclusively upon private promotion and sale of a product. It is not clear just how this public policy has developed. It may have been the wish of the pharmaceutical companies that there be no public support. It may have been the public opinion that pharmacy dealt solely in a product which would be sold at a profit and that it was inappropriate to use tax funds.

The nature of pharmacy has been substantially affected by the circumstances described above. The amount of research and development is obviously determined by the earnings of the industry. If earnings decline, the amount of research must also decline. As inflation and increasing governmental regulation augment the cost of developing and bringing a new drug to market, the number of new drugs produced will decrease. Further, since profits finance research, the areas investigated and emphasized will be those which are most likely to be profitable. No pharmaceutical company could afford to develop a new drug for the cure of a disease or condition found in only 10,000 patients each year and whose cure could be effected with the administration of a few doses of the drug. A new drug to deal with a very common and chronic condition, such as hypertension, will have very large and long-continuing sales and hence will be profitable. These observations are not made in criticism of either public policy or of the pharmaceutical manufacturers. They are made to point out that there are some ways in which pharmacy is different and has some unique problems. The way in which these problems are addressed and eventually solved will have a profound effect upon pharmacy and pharmacists, upon patients, and upon the public.

VI. PHARMACY'S INFORMATION SYSTEM

In Chapter II we have advanced the concept that pharmacy is best described and defined as a *knowledge system*. If this concept is valid some ultimate judgments concerning the field must be made in terms of how it deals with knowledge and information, or fails to do so. We have already dealt with how knowledge is developed in pharmacy through research and from access to the basic sciences and other disciplines such as medicine. It is obvious how a part of that knowledge is translated into a drug product through the steps of development and manufacturing. It is also clear how the portion of the knowledge encapsulated in the drug product is ultimately delivered to the patient. What happens to the balance of the knowledge is not so obvious.

The knowledge and information of pharmacy is complex and confusing. It is complex because it deals *with drugs and with people*. Drugs are complex chemical substances with complex pharmacological properties. To understand them, their structure, and their properties requires a high degree of chemical and pharmacological knowledge and sophistication. People are even more complex than chemicals or drugs. The effect of a given drug dosage upon a patient is by no means always predictable. Drugs do not dissolve at the same rate; they are not absorbed into the blood stream at the same rate; they are not metabolized at the same rate; they are not excreted at the same rate in all individuals. Some individuals are allergic to certain drugs. The state of health or of disease of the individual has a profound effect upon the pharmacological and physiological effects of a given drug. Beyond these differences there are complexities which arise from psychological, cultural, and social factors. Diet, exercise, the use of alcohol, all can and do alter the pharmacological effects of drugs in individual patients. Some individuals seem to believe that there is a pill for every disease, pain, discomfort or mood. They virtually demand that the physician prescribe a drug for every ailment real or imagined. They consume quantities of OTC drugs. Understanding such an individual and his total interaction with drugs in health and in episodes of disease requires a vast store of physical, biological, and behavioral knowledge.

Pharmacy knowledge and information is confusing because there are tens of thousands of drugs or drug products available. Most of them appear on the market with a copyrighted trade name. Thus, there may be many identical or closely similar products from which the prescribing physician must choose. Identical drugs appear in multiple dosage forms. Combinations of several drugs appear in separate formulations. Many OTC drugs are proprietary formulations. The task of knowing the chemical, pharmacological, physiological, and kinetic properties of all drug products clearly taxes the power of even the most highly educated of professionals.

There are three groups of people who need the knowledge and information of pharmacy. First, there are the physicians who must choose and prescribe a drug therapy and those who work with them to provide patient care such as nurses and other therapists; second, there are the pharmacists who must dispense; third, there are the patients who consume or utilize drugs. A part of the education of the physician is in the field of pharmacology and pharmacotherapeutics. In this education future physicians receive knowledge and information about drugs, about their actions, their adverse reactions, their effect upon various disease states, and about the possible idiosyncrasies in individual patients. It is believed by some medical educators that the physician is properly prepared to decide upon a drug therapy for each of his patients and to prescribe the proper drug and drug regimen. Other medical educators have observed that not enough attention is given to drugs and drug therapy in physician education, inasmuch as the extent of knowledge has grown very rapidly and the complexity of drug therapy has increased. All are agreed that the knowledge and information about drugs gained during formal education becomes rapidly obsolete. New drugs are constantly introduced, new therapies are put into practice, adverse reactions are identified. It is said that ninety percent of the drugs currently in use were not available at the time when many practicing physicians were receiving their education. Thus, the system or mechanism by which physicians month after month and year after year obtain a continuing flow of knowledge and information about drugs and drug therapy is of great import to the maintenance of high standards of drug therapy and its prescription.

Physicians obtain drug information in a variety of ways. There are many articles on drugs and drug therapy in the professional journals. The same journals carry many advertisements of the pharmaceutical manufacturers. There are several pharmacopoeias, the *Physician's Desk Reference,* hospital formularies available and usually at hand for reference. The pharmacopoeias are voluminous tomes recording complex data on a host of drugs. They are revised and updated at intervals. However, they cannot keep up with all of the new drugs constantly appearing and the new clinical findings on old drugs flowing from continuing reports of physician and patient experience. Thus, the pharmacopoeias are never complete. The *Physician's Desk Reference* is that most frequently consulted by prescribing physicians. It, however, is not a complete reference work for it contains only the material furnished at the time of annual publication by the manufacturer of the drug product and is no more complete than a package insert. Further, the manufacturer pays for the inclusion of information about his products. Thus, some products may not appear in the volume. By regulation the manufacturer must include a package insert which carries information useful to the physician contemplating the use of a particular drug. The physician is visited by representatives of the pharmaceutical manufacturers (detail men) who provide him with information about the drugs marketed by that particular manufacturer. The oral presentation is frequently supplemented by brochures, reprints, and other visual material.

Finally, the physician obtains drug information through consultation; most frequently he consults his clinical colleagues. In some situations he is able to consult a drug therapy specialist—the clinical pharmacologist. In hospital practice the physician may consult the institution's pharmacy staff. In what appears to be a rare event he may consult a retail pharmacist. There have been a few studies of how and from whom physicians obtain drug information. The results show that the most frequently used sources are colleagues, textbooks and journals, compendia, and detail men. However, the nature of the physician's practice may have a substantial effect upon the sources from which he obtains his drug information. The physician in solo practice is likely to depend more heavily upon detail men for he sees his colleagues with less frequency and access to complete library facilities may be difficult. The hospital physician consults with colleagues frequently and depends far less upon seeing detail men. The least frequently used source of information is consultation with a pharmacist.

Physicians do obtain information about drugs continually from many sources. However, two observations must be made. First, there is no organized system for knowledge acquisition. What is available has developed haphazardly and without rational planning. Second, there is no mechanism for determining the accuracy and validity of some of the information available; presumably that carried by a scholarly article in a well-refereed scientific journal should be complete and highly reliable. The same cannot be said for all the advertisements of drug manufacturers or all the presentations of detail men. The value of consultation with a colleague is wholly dependent on the competence of that colleague.

The transmission of knowledge and information to the pharmacist resembles in part and differs in part from that to the physician. The knowledge that has gone into the development and the manufacturing of drugs is an important part of the formal education of the pharmacist. He learns about the chemistry, biology, physics, pharmacology of drugs, and their effects. He also learns some of the knowledge of pharmacy that does not go into the production of the drug. He learns about absorption, metabolism, kinetics, interactions, and adverse reactions.

The pharmacist has the same need for updated information as does the physician. As many as ninety percent of the drugs he dispenses may not have been invented or on the market at the time of his formal education. Although the information need of the pharmacist is as urgent as that of the physician, his access to that information is substantially less. Scholarly articles on new drugs are carried by the relatively few professional pharmacy journals and there are brief items in news sheets. Pharmacists can and do read the package inserts provided by drug manufacturers for physicians; however, they are not regularly visited by detail men. They have access to pharmacopoeias, formularies, and reference books. Pharmacies are required by law to have the *National Formulary* and the *United States Pharmacopoeia.* However, other important reference sources are not as readily available to pharmacists as they should be. A pharmacist can consult colleagues, but this is difficult unless he is working with other pharmacists such as in a large hospital situation. There is perhaps one way in which a pharmacist's access to information may be better than that of a physician; this is in the area of continuing education courses and materials. Continuing education for physicians contains drug information but only as a small proportion of the total knowledge conveyed. Continuing education of pharmacists contains drug information as its major component.

Again, one must observe that there is no convenient, easily accessible, and highly reliable information *system* available to the pharmacist. He must depend on a variety of sources and their availability. It may well take a dedicated professional to keep as up to date as he should.

There have been some attempts to provide better drug information services to physicians, nurses, and pharmacists. As mentioned before, drug information centers have been set up in many cities and in a growing number of hospitals and medical centers. However, the number is not increasing and in fact is falling. The utilization of such centers by physicians and pharmacists has not been as great as might be expected. Further, they have proved expensive. Costs of ten to twenty dollars per question answered have been reported. It is difficult to explain these facts. Physicians, nurses, and pharmacists state that they need more information, but they do not utilize drug information centers with any frequency. There are probably many reasons for this paradox; it may be that the cost is too high; it may be that the centers have not been properly conceived, located, and set up; it may be that the centers have not made proper use of new information technology and hardware. The Study Commission does call attention to the drug information problem. We suggest that some agency, association, bureau, or foundation might devote major attention to the problem and find out who needs to know, what he needs to know, and how those needs can best be met with speed and economy.

The need for accurate and useful drug information by the ultimate user of drug products—the patient—is infrequently considered. There is no organized way in which such information is made available. The education received by laymen rarely includes anything about drugs. Mass media contain few informational items, but much drug advertising and promotion. Physicians do give instructions concerning the administration of drugs to the patient along with a prescription. Nurses do give some further instructions to patients leaving a hospital. Public health nurses provide surveillance of drug therapy for patients in their homes. Some pharmacists endeavor to re-inforce physician instructions and describe expected results from the medi-cations they dispense. Still, there is evidence that the vast majority of pa-tients need more information. Studies of how patients use medicine show that less than half of all prescriptions are followed completely. Patients make errors in the amount and frequency of dosage; they fail to complete the total regimen ordered; they even do not get some prescriptions filled; they take prescription drugs ordered for another member of the family. Studies of the sources from which patients get drug advice indicate that family, friends, and neighbors are the most frequent source. Physicians and mass media advertising follow and pharmacists are named last. *It is no won-der that many Americans are overusers and misusers of drugs.*

The information needs of the public are numerous and complex. The pa-tient will never use a drug information center, nor is he likely to frequently consult physicians or pharmacists. Some kind of mass communication is in-dicated; some kind of consumer education must be developed. However, much can be done by physicians, nurses, the drug industry, and particularly by pharmacists. There must be some changes in habits of practice; some changes in methods of compensation, and much greater communication be-tween health professionals.

It has been stated that there is no effective drug information system. It should be added that the system of pharmacy has some circumstances which impede the flow of information and which make full communication extremely difficult. The first of these circumstances arises from the propri-etary nature of much drug knowledge. The knowledge is acquired under proprietary auspices and is properly owned by the corporation which pays for its acquisition. Knowledge not paid for by the public comes slowly into the public domain. True, in order to obtain approval from the FDA to market a new drug, a pharmaceutical manufacturer must provide that agency with huge amounts of data and clinical evidence; but this does not put all of the knowledge immediately into the public domain. It does get there piece by piece but it takes time. A second circumstance affecting the free flow of in-formation is the gap between the compounding part and the dispensing part of pharmacy. The two parts are articulated to distribute drug products, not to distribute drug information. If the product moves from the manufacturer to the retailer through a wholesaler there is another gap in the information chain. A third circumstance arises from the fact that the physician is abso-lutely essential to the process of getting the proper drug to the patient at the right time, but he is not in the system of pharmacy. Without a prescription there can be no dispensing. Yet, the drug product does not pass from manu-facturer to the pharmacist through the physician. Thus, there is a gap in communication. The manufacturer may communicate with the physician and he may communicate with the pharmacist but not through the physician. To say it simply, pharmacists and physicians do not communicate very often, and if they do it is in spite of the system not because of it.

One further observation about drug knowledge and information needs to be made. There is a widely held impression that there is an abundance of drug knowledge and information and that if only it could be pried out of manufacturers, the FDA, and specialists and put into an effective and accessible system every conceivable drug question could be answered. The data on the clinical testing of a new drug do answer some questions about what *did* happen under carefully controlled situations involving selected patients and specially skilled physicians. The data do not answer questions about what *will* happen under uncontrolled conditions involving unselected patients and physicians having wide variation in training and experience. Pharmacy is not yet an exact science; it still is partly pragmatic. A better information system will improve pharmacy, but it will not solve all drug-related problems. There is still much to be learned and our national policy in the support of drug research needs careful examination.

However, there is much information which is not used and the system could be improved even though there are large gaps in knowledge. One can conceive procedures for obtaining a systematic feedback into the health information system concerning the actual experiences which patients have with the drugs prescribed, including whether they are taken according to directions and the appearance of both desirable and undesirable effects. With such information feedback, the pharmacist could provide much data about drug efficacy and drug utilization which is not now gathered but which surely would result in improved drug therapy,

The Study Commission believes that the system of pharmacy must be described as being both effective and efficient in developing, manufacturing, and distributing drug products. A wide variety of drugs is conveniently available to those who require them throughout the nation in cities, towns, and rural areas. However, the system of pharmacy cannot be described as either effective or efficient in developing, organizing, and distributing knowledge and information about drugs. When pharmacy is viewed as a knowledge system, it must be judged as only partially successful in delivering its full potential as a health service to the members of society.

VII. FORCES OF CHANGE IN HEALTH SERVICES: IMPLICATIONS FOR PHARMACY

The past twenty-five years have seen rapid and very extensive change in health services in the United States. These changes have come about in response to forces both internal and external to the health professions. The forces are scientific, technological, social, economic, and political. The resulting changes have affected pharmacy and its practitioners and will continue to affect them in the foreseeable future. In this chapter we shall endeavor to review the forces and changes and to describe the implications, both present and future, to pharmacy and pharmacists.

The most dramatic change has occurred in society's views and attitudes concerning the utility of health services. The first fifty years of the twentieth century clearly demonstrated that public health measures, the services of physicians and other health workers, and ever more powerful drugs could and did produce dramatic effects upon mortality and morbidity, upon life expectancy, and upon the well-being and comfort of the people who received them. Access to health services, which was earlier regarded as a privilege, came to be viewed as a necessity and now as a right of every citizen. To enjoy such a right there must be no barriers—financial or geographic—to obtaining it. Society has therefore become concerned with removing financial barriers to health services and with ensuring access to all citizens. The public concern has more recently extended itself to the question of quality of health services with legislation requiring accountability from those providing them and mandating regional planning for health services.

During this century scientific research has provided more effective medical technology—sophisticated surgical procedures, antibiotics and other powerful drugs, more effective diagnostic tools. The capacity of health professionals to cope with episodes of severe illness has been enhanced. Knowledge has been obtained that makes it possible not only to cure illness but in some cases to prevent it or to control the processes which lead to episodes of illness. The improvement in sanitation and nutrition has resulted in the control of the incidence of some disease with a resulting decrease in morbidity and mortality. The approach to some categories of disease, notably those of infectious nature, has shifted from one of care and cure to one of prevention.

Society has reacted to these internal changes by asking for greater comprehensiveness and continuity of health services. Our citizens are asking not only for the cure of episodes of illness but also for services to assure the maintenance of health and the prevention of disease. This desire and demand are seen in the expectation that the health services system will encompass additional responsibilities such as dealing with the health problems of alcoholism, drug abuse, obesity, and emotional distress.

Most recently society has become deeply concerned with the cost of health services. As a nation we have come to the realization that our resources are not limitless and that ultimately we must decide how much we can afford to devote to medical and health care. At the same time newer and more powerful medical technologies, such as heart surgery, renal dialysis, and psychotropic drugs, are being utilized; and they are extremely expensive. It is natural that we now have great concern for the efficiency achieved in the delivery of all health services. It is likely that we shall find that we cannot afford all the health services we wish or are possible.

These forces of change have altered the health services delivery system in regard to financing, demand, organization, control, character, and the communication of information.

Financing

Historically personal medical care has been paid for by the individual receiving it, by private philanthropy, or by tax funds on behalf of those on public welfare. The federal government has in recent decades assumed financial responsibility for the health care needs of an ever-growing segment of the population. The government has long been responsible for medical care of members of the armed forces, for veterans, and for some other groups such as maritime workers. In the last quarter century other groups of citizens have been added to these responsibilities—senior citizens through Medicare and the medically indigent through Medicaid. During the same time period the concept of health insurance through voluntary and private mechanisms has grown remarkably. Millions of citizens are now enrolled in Blue Cross and Blue Shield programs. Millions of workers have obtained health insurance protection as a fringe benefit in union contracts. Other millions of citizens have developed programs to provide and to pay for medical and hospital services through health maintenance organizations, medical foundations, and consumer-owned cooperatives. As a result, the vast majority of American citizens, perhaps as many as ninety percent, have the costs of their health care paid for in full or in part by third parties operated either by government or by private agencies. Physician fees, hospital bills, and prescription drugs are more and more frequently paid for, at least in part, by someone other than the patient receiving the service. Now we, as a nation, are discussing the concept of a national health insurance program which would include every citizen and cover the costs of most, if not all, health services required. Most observers agree that the United States will have such a program and in the near future. Thus, we are at—or nearing—the time when financial barriers to the access to services will be removed for all Americans.

Demand

The removal of financial barriers has already resulted in a great increase in demand for health services of all kinds. The number of visits to physicians, the number of hospitalizations, the number of drug prescriptions have all increased markedly. In spite of a rapid growth in the number of practicing physicians and other health professionals there are geographic areas which are unserved or underserved and in which people do not have access to health services which they desire. The shortage of primary care facilities seems of particular concern. There is evidence of a shortage of professional health care services to patients in nursing homes and in mental hospitals which has led to inferior standards of care and some undesirable practices such as the overprescribing of drugs. When a national health insurance program is established we must expect a further escalation in demand. Thus, manpower and facilities will be called upon to serve even more patients. Demographic changes will have an additional impact. Based upon the currently reasonable assumption of a fertility rate of 2.1 births per woman, the Census Bureau projects that the total United States population will rise from 211,909,000 in 1974 to 262,494,999 in the year 2000.[4] The predicted increase in the number of persons sixty years of age and older is from 31,010,00 [*sic*] in 1974 to 40,590,000 in the year 2000. The percentage increase in the total population for the period is 23.9; for the members sixty years and older it is 30.9. The population group which requires a disproportionately large amount of medical and health care is increasing most rapidly. We must look forward to an increasing demand in the health field for years to come.

Organization and Institutionalization

The past three or four decades have seen an ever-increasing amount of organization and institutionalization in the delivery of health services. Some advances in medical technology require that more and more patients be hospitalized in order to have the full benefit of those advances. The hospital has become the focus of medical activities and the locus for the practice of many specialties. In turn, hospitals, in a sense, have become parts of a system in which there are different kinds of institutions to care for patients with varying degrees of need for services of special competence. Frequently hospitals are described as being primary, secondary, or tertiary care facilities. As convalescent facilities and intermediate and long-term care institutions have developed, health services have been further institutionalized. The result has been that a growing number of patients are receiving their care not from a single health professional but from a group of health workers, many of whom are employees of institutions. To many of our citizens the hospital and not the physician is seen as the principal source of medical services. The rapid growth of the usage of the hospital emergency room as a place to obtain all sorts of care for chronic and for episodic illness is evidence of this aspect of institutionalization.

Medical practice has become increasingly organized. Growing knowledge demands specialization. Specialization requires a division of labor which in turn demands organization. The group practice of medicine has grown rapidly. Physicians have formed organizations of several kinds: there are multispecialty groups; there are single specialty groups; there are many varieties of clinics; there are medical care foundations; there are prepaid systems employing physicians. There are probably many reasons for the increased organization of physicians: they desire a more controllable work schedule; they desire the opportunity for rapid and frequent consultation.

However, the most powerful force toward this accelerated organization is the need for added efficiency as a means to respond to a growing demand for medical service. Organization does make possible more efficient utilization of the physician's time. It gives the opportunity to employ various kinds of assistants and associates and to utilize knowledge and skills possessed by members of other professions and vocations. Group and institutional practice does make possible the introduction of the "health team" concept. Potentially, at least, the team concept does give promise for greater productivity and possibly for reduced cost. There can be no doubt that the degree of organization is growing. There are regions where group practice is almost universal. The forces which have brought this about are not abating. Actually they are increasing and we must expect further organization and additional institutionalization.

An additional force encouraging organization is the inevitable consequence of the rise of the importance of third-party payers for health services. Patients are enrolled in a wide variety of health care plans. Each of these plans specifies the health services which are to be provided or paid for. To care for these patients all health professionals, hospitals, and nursing homes must adapt and accept some of the consequences of increasing organization and institutionalization.

Quality Control

With the rapid rise of federal participation in financing health care costs, with the rise in the popularity of health insurance, with the appearance of various kinds of HMOs, with the initiation of medical foundations and consumer-owned health care cooperatives has come a concern for the quality of the services to be provided. It is unlikely that a governmental agency, a private insurance company, or voluntary subscribers to a prepaid health service program would contract to pay for services without specifying in advance the character, the amount, and the standards of those services; nor is it likely that a society would decide that health care was a basic human right without demanding that the care provided meet a minimum standard of quality. The earliest attempts to set standards of quality took the form of specifying the services for which compensation would be paid. A more elaborate and sophisticated system is beginning to appear in the implementation of federal legislation mandating professional standards review organizations (PSROs). Hospital utilization, length of stay, surgical procedures, drug utilization, and patient outcomes will be examined, monitored, and judged. In the process standards of care will be developed, institutional governance examined, mechanisms of control devised. Society is concerned with the questions of quality and of cost and is asking for accountability on the part of health care providers. The current concern about nursing home inadequacies is an example of the public expectation for quality assurance. Legislation at the state and the national level will ensue; standards will be set and review mechanisms created.

Cost Containment

As a nation we are faced with a dilemma. On the one hand, we accept the concept that access to health services is a necessity and a right. We are moving steadily toward a goal of removing all economic barriers to such access for all of our citizens. We have seen that this policy has resulted in a much greater demand for and utilization of resources of all kinds. We must be prepared for further increases in demand and utilization when fiscal barriers are further reduced or totally eliminated. The national cost of providing health services has risen spectacularly because of growing demand, new modalities of treatment, and because of inflation. On the other hand, we have belatedly come to the realization that our national resources are not unlimited and that there is a ceiling upon the amount of money, manpower, and facilities which we can afford to devote to health.

In facing the dilemma attention has turned to finding ways to contain the costs of providing health services. Each piece of legislation which has extended the federal responsibility for the costs of health care to particular groups of citizens has contained regulations concerning services to be provided and setting maximum costs of such services which would be reimbursed. Every private insurance program carries the same kind of definition of services to be provided and/or limitation of costs to be reimbursed. Every prepaid plan specifies services and requires subscriber payments determined by the predicted costs of those services. Thus, much of the health service system of today operates under a variety of cost containment regulations. If and when a national health insurance program is enacted, it will surely provide for vigorous cost controls.

The health services delivery system has been affected by these economic facts. It will be further affected in the future. It is clear that the review mechanisms mandated under PSRO legislation are, or will be, charged not only with monitoring and controlling quality of services but also with monitoring and controlling costs. Hospital admissions, length of hospital stays, use of prescription drugs, surgical procedures, and laboratory tests will be monitored. All health workers, all health service providing institutions will be involved and directly affected.

One cannot predict with accuracy just how the health services delivery system will react to an ever more stringent cost containment program. However one reaction will be to try to find ways and means of increasing efficiency as a means of containing or reducing costs. Such attempts will certainly result in further division of labor, increased organization, and greater institutionalization. More and more health care will be provided by organized groups of health workers or by institutions employing health workers. Thus, the force of cost containment will reinforce the changes already in progress.

Primary Care

One area of health service which is receiving great attention under the necessity imposed by fiscal restraints and as a consequence of concepts of improved health care is that frequently referred to as "primary care." There is not yet complete agreement on either the words or their meaning. In general the reference is to those health services required by patients who are suffering from minor injury, from self-limiting disease, from controllable disease processes, from irreversible chronic disease. Sometimes the expression "ambulatory care" is used since most of the required services can be provided on an ambulatory basis and do not require hospital facilities. That term, however, does not include extended nursing home care which involves few patients who are truly ambulatory. The objection to the rise of the word "primary" to describe this kind of health service arises from the conflict with its use in describing the "primary physician." A primary physician is generally regarded as one who is primarily and continuously responsible for a patient's diagnosis and treatment whether his needs of the moment demand primary, secondary, tertiary, or preventive care. Suffice it to say that all observers agree that there is an area of health service which should be organized to deliver less elaborate and less costly care than is required for the drastically ill patient who must have specialist medical care and the use of costly institutional facilities and procedures. It must be expected that we shall see the development of a variety of organizations, institutions, and programs to provide these services with greater efficiency and quality and with less cost.

In the changes which lie ahead hospitals will alter or extend their activities. New kinds of institutions will appear; new uses of auxiliary personnel will be made; different working relations between health professionals will be worked out; professional practice will change as well as practice environments; new links between services of various complexity and sophistication will be forged.

The Right to Know

In addition to all of the internal and external forces which are producing change in the health services delivery system and which have been discussed above, there is an additional social force which has arisen and which promises to grow in influence. This force may best be described as the "right to know." As organized society has begun to participate more actively in determining philosophies and programs in the area of health, as our citizens have become better informed and more concerned, we see demands for lay participation in many aspects of health services. We see this in the consumer movement. We see this in the appearance of ombudsmen or patient advocates in our hospitals. We see this in the requirements for lay participation in health planning of many kinds. Basically, this arises from a desire on the part of the public for more information. Historically the health professions have not been too deeply concerned about providing knowledge and information to those whom they serve. Medicine is a descendant of witchcraft and the priestly function. For centuries it has had a certain aura of secrecy and a cloak of exclusivity of knowledge. It has been viewed as doing something to or for the patient who is the passive and unenlightened recipient of a benefit he could not obtain otherwise. Concepts are changing; information is being requested; public participation is being demanded.

Again we see a force which is growing and will in the future grow in magnitude. The health service delivery system will respond in the only way possible; that way is to become not only a service provider but an information provider as well. This will require more effective communication between professionals and patients. Particularly it will require more effective communication between health professionals of all kinds. The provision for such communication will require new interprofessional cooperation and collaboration. It will require the utilization of new information systems; it will require the installation of sophisticated information handling technology; it will require alterations in the education of health professionals so that they may not only transmit skill but also appropriate knowledge and information.

Unmet Needs

There is a *potential* force of change in health services which must be described. This potential force arises because there are some identifiable unmet needs in the drug therapy provided to patients. If these needs are met with the active participation of pharmacists, there will be a strong factor of change operating upon pharmacy practice.

A number of perceptive physicians, pharmacists, and scientists have pointed out an important gap in the health care system concerning the development, dissemination, and utilization of knowledge and skills in the areas of pharmacokinetics (including bioavailability, the influence of disease on the fate of drugs in the body, interindividual variability), individualization of the dosage of a drug, drug interactions, and adverse drug reactions. They recognize that while physicians may know about the action of drugs on the body, the physicians are not knowledgeable about the fate of drugs in the body which, of course, influences the action of drugs.

Some hospital administrators have observed that while surgical therapy and radiation therapy are well organized and run smoothly in their institutions, drug therapy is not well organized and responsibility of the several professional groups is not clearly defined. Some nurses have observed that there are serious gaps in the nurses' knowledge of drug therapy and particularly in the communication of needed drug information to their patients.

One must conclude from these observations of practicing health professionals that there are serious gaps in the drug therapy portion of the health care system. Further, it must be expected that with a rising demand for improved quality of health care there will be efforts to fill these gaps and to meet the identified needs.

Implications for Pharmacy

Pharmacy is one of the health services and it is therefore affected by all of the forces which are producing change in the health services system. The response of pharmacy to these forces will in some instances be similar to those of other parts of the system. In some instances the response of pharmacy will be unique. We are at a period in our national history when the character, the magnitude, and the direction of some of the forces can be determined and evaluated. Thus, it is possible to predict with some hope of accuracy the changes in pharmacy which will develop in response to the several forces. In the following paragraphs the Study Commission will present its views upon the changes which can be expected to arise in relation to pharmacy.

Financing

The pattern of financing of health services is now clearly established. Third-party payment is rapidly becoming the norm for payment for services and for health related products. Already many prescriptions are paid for by government programs, by insurance benefits, by prepaid service programs. A few pharmacists have taken the step of initiating programs for the prepayment of prescription drugs. A national health insurance program is certain to include payments, in whole or in part, for prescription drugs. The historical arrangement whereby the patient or client pays the pharmacist directly for the drug dispensed will begin to disappear, to be replaced by a system in which the dispensing pharmacist is paid by a third party.

Such a development in the payment system will demand changes in pharmacy practice. The dispensing pharmacist will be forced to more elaborate record keeping. He will be forced to provide more extensive data. This in turn will require the use of more efficient information technology. It is safe to predict that the pharmacist will come more and more to depend upon the computer as a constantly used tool of his practice and at the same time will find available to him more knowledge that will have significance for health care.

It is likely that the change in financing will accelerate the shift away from the markup on the cost of a drug product to compensate the pharmacist for his dispensing service to the use of a dispensing fee. Retainer fees, consultation fees, capitation fees are other possibilities particularly in prepaid plans and in extended care facilities. This shift will enable the pharmacist to evaluate the costs of his services and will provide the opportunity to define those services more accurately and expand them.

Demand

The growth in demand for health services of all kinds will be felt in the profession of pharmacy. A substantial majority of therapeutic services and many currently used preventive services involve drug products. Many authorities predict that when national health insurance is operative we shall see the number of prescriptions rise from three and a half billion per year to five or perhaps six billion. Further, the progress of medical technology may be in the direction of increased drug utilization. In conquering tuberculosis, hospitalization and lung surgery have been replaced by drug therapy. In conquering polio, long hospitalization and physical therapy have been replaced by immunization. In the area of mental disease, long-time custodial hospitalization and shock treatment are being replaced with an ever-increasing use of psychotropic drugs. It is probably fair to say that the impact of growing demand will be felt most sharply in the area of pharmacy services.

It is clear that pharmacy and pharmacists must find ways to meet a greatly expanded demand and with the expectation that the number of pharmacists will grow less rapidly than demand. It is imperative that the efficiency of the process by which prescription drugs are dispensed rise by a factor of probably one hundred percent. This is true for all dispensing pharmacists whether they practice in community, hospital, clinic, or nursing home environments. Such an increase in efficiency will be possible only by exploiting every opportunity for mechanization and automation for the performance of routine and nonprofessional tasks. It will require the use of larger numbers of less well-trained workers in technical and clerical roles. The future will not permit the use of the full-trained pharmacist in procedures and tasks that do not require the level of his knowledge and skill.

Organization and Institutionalization

As the hospital has become more and more the focus of medical services, an increasing portion of pharmacy has moved into the hospital. Hospital pharmacy is today the fastest growing segment of the profession. As the care of patients with chronic disease and disability has moved into the nursing home, pharmacy has developed special means for meeting the drug requirements of those patients. As new forms of health services delivery have developed, pharmacy and pharmacists have moved into those institutions. As further institutionalization occurs more pharmacy will be institutionalized and more pharmacists will be employed in that environment.

However, one cannot visualize a time when all of pharmacy dispensing will be within health care institutions. In the first place, institutions are neither the most economical nor the most acceptable arrangements for the delivery of all health services. Some services are best and most economically provided in other arrangements such as a doctor's office or in the home by a visiting nurse. Second, there is a countervailing force which is particularly significant to pharmacy; that force is the need and the public desire for availability and accessibility. Pharmacy has been and is the most accessible of the health services because of the broad distribution of pharmacies. Pharmacists are more available than physicians; pharmacies are more available than hospitals or clinics.

The resolution of the two forces—the need for institutionalization for greater efficiency and the need for availability—demands a form of organization as an alternative to institutionalization. It is possible to gain the benefits of organization without institutionalizing in the physical sense. Pharmacists have already begun to organize cooperative associations for purchasing. Such cooperatives can be expanded for other services such as record keeping, drug utilization data, and management services. It can be visualized that all the community pharmacists in a geographic area could be a part of an information and communication network through the exploitation of present and future technology. It is surely possible to improve the communication between pharmacists and physicians without having to place them side by side physically and within the walls of a single institution.

The trends of the future seem clear. More pharmacists will practice in institutions; probably fewer will be individual entrepreneurs. All pharmacists, whatever their practice environment, will become more and more a part of a system not only of pharmacy but of health services as a whole. Finally, the pharmacists will practice differently; they will have and use more sophisticated tools; and they will be assisted by a growing number of technical workers.

Quality Control

Pharmacy cannot be left out of the mechanism developing for the setting of standards for and the monitoring of health services. Drug therapy is a major part of health care and pharmacy is a part of drug therapy. Thus PSROs will be responsible for peer review of drug prescribing, drug utilization, drug efficacy and safety, and patient outcomes. The pharmacist should be particularly involved in monitoring drug utilization. He must therefore be a part of the PSRO. A beginning has been made in some hospitals, in several prepaid health services systems, and in at least one voluntary system. As quality control becomes widespread pharmacists will find themselves involved. They will be asked to set standards of pharmacy services; they will be asked to monitor drug utilization; they may be asked to concern themselves with patients' compliance and experiences with adverse drug reactions.

Cost Containment

In 1975 efforts to contain costs of health services include an active public concern about the costs of drugs. There are conflicting data about the trends of drug costs. Per capita annual expenditures for out-of-hospital prescriptions rose from $6.85 in 1950 to $16.05 in 1966. In that same period the number of prescriptions per individual rose from 2.4 per annum to 4.6. Drug expenditures accounted for 11.7 percent of all health expenditures in 1957 but accounted for only 9.8 percent in 1966.[5] Further, many new and more powerful drugs came on the market during that period which, although commanding a higher price per dosage unit, may have proved more efficacious and thus required fewer dosages per illness. The debate about drug prices will continue nevertheless. There is the expectation of growing governmental regulation such as a policy mandating generic prescribing. Medicare, Medicaid, and many private insurance programs carry maximum allowable reimbursements for drugs dispensed. National health insurance will surely contain regulation of costs of both products and services.

In view of these prospects, it behooves pharmacists to take immediate steps to define their services, to determine their costs, to be prepared to enter into those mechanisms which will set standards and monitor performance. PSROs will surely become mechanisms for both quality assurance and for cost containment.

Primary Care

Pharmacy is an important part of the activity popularly known as "primary care" which was described earlier in this chapter. Most of the patients it serves are ambulatory. The therapy provided to patients suffering from minor illness and to chronically ill patients involves drugs, particularly prescription drugs. Probably the largest segment of "primary care" is self-care, and self-care frequently involves self-medication. The pharmacist is probably the only health worker who can influence this part of primary care, since many nonprescription drugs are bought in community pharmacies. The final form that primary care will take is not wholly clear. It is certain that such care will receive much attention from both the professions and the public. It is to the interest of pharmacy and pharmacists that they be active in conceiving, testing, and implementing organizations, techniques, and procedures to achieve an efficient, high quality, and economical system. Perhaps this is a problem for scholarly inquiry and study to which the colleges of pharmacy should devote themselves with vigor and dispatch.

The Right to Know

Nowhere in the health services system is the right, the need, the demand to know more apparent than in pharmacy. And, one must add, nowhere in the health services system is there less provision for meeting that right, that need, and that demand. Pharmacy is a generally excellent system for generating knowledge, for translating knowledge into a product, for distributing the product, and for dispensing the product; but it is far from an excellent system for transmitting knowledge and information, particularly to the ultimate consumer—the patient. It strikes some observers as ironic that the pharmaceutical industry, which is one of the most highly developed from a scientific and technological point of view, should in part disseminate its knowledge to physicians by a one-to-one interview between a detail man and a single physician. It almost seems like using the pony express in a day of instant electronic communication. Communication to the pharmacist is scanty and not well organized. Communication between physician and pharmacist is spotty and incomplete. (It is no wonder that no provision has been made for the public's need for information.)

There is much evidence that knowledge and perspective about drugs must be greatly increased for all people. We are a nation of drug takers; some of us have become drug abusers. Many of us consume drugs for which we have no need because we are persuaded by advertising or the advice of neighbors and friends. Most important, drug therapy inevitably and very frequently involves the patient and his personal decisions. A diagnosis may be made with the greatest of skill, a regimen of drug therapy may be carefully prescribed, the prescription may be accurately dispensed, but the patient may make any one of a number of decisions which negates the whole process. He may decide not to buy the drug; he may decide to take more or less than prescribed; he may decide to discontinue the drug before the regimen has been concluded; he may take it with another substance, drug, or food which will neutralize the first drug or produce an adverse reaction. Since the patient, in a very real sense, makes the ultimate decision at the very least it ought to be an informed decision; but an informed decision can only be based on adequate information. Thus, we again express the opinion that the greatest failing of pharmacy is its inadequacy as an information transmitting system.

Pharmacists can do something to improve the transmission of knowledge. First, they can acquire knowledge themselves. Second, they can communicate with physicians and other health professionals. Third, they can communicate with patients. Fourth, they can join others in developing a mechanism whereby drug information is widely disseminated through all the mass media. Fifth, pharmacists can enter into an effective drug information system using the most advanced technology.

Unmet Needs

Unmet needs in the area of drug therapy have been identified as an added *potential* force acting to produce change in the practice of pharmacy. There is no doubt that there are gaps. Drug therapy can be improved in a number of ways for it does fall short of providing the optimal benefit to patients. It is highly likely that steps will be taken to close the gap between the optimal and the actual. The important question is what part will pharmacy and pharmacists play? Pharmacists are presumed to have expert knowledge about pharmacokinetics, bioavailability, dosage individualization and the interindividual variability of response to drug therapy. In a number of ways the pharmacist should be more knowledgeable in these areas than is the physician. The pharmacist generally is not now expert in the field of human behavior which must have a great deal to do with patient compliance. There is at the present no great demand that pharmacists assume leadership in fulfilling unmet needs. However, the Study Commission wishes to stress the point that in this area lies a great opportunity for pharmacy and pharmacists. If they can contribute constructively, if they can demonstrate superior knowledge and skill, other health professionals and society as a whole will welcome the development of new and more demanding roles for pharmacists.

VIII. FORCES OF CHANGE INTERNAL TO PHARMACY

Not only are the system of pharmacy and the practice of pharmacists of all kinds responding to economic, social, and political changes and to changes in the health care delivery system, but they are also responding to forces of change which are internal to pharmacy itself. These internal forces are not operating in a single direction and toward a single end. They are diverse in character as well as direction.

Pharmacy is a profession composed of numerous groups representing specific interests and diverse points of view. If one defines a profession as "the body of those who practice a particular art or vocation," one has some difficulty in identifying the profession of pharmacy. There are a surprising number of associations and groups of pharmacists, the largest and most active of which are:

1. *The American Pharmaceutical Association,* in which approximately one-half of the registered pharmacists of the country hold individual membership.
2. *The National Association of Retail Druggists,* which includes a majority of owners of independent community pharmacies. This organization at one time was a section of APhA.
3. *The American Society of Hospital Pharmacists,* which includes a majority of the pharmacists practicing in hospitals and other patient care institutions. It, too, was once a section of the APhA.
4. *The National Association of Chain Drug Stores,* in which corporations operating four or more retail pharmacies hold membership.
5. *The Pharmaceutical Manufacturers Association,* in which nearly all drug manufacturing companies hold membership.
6. *The Academy of Pharmaceutical Sciences,* in which pharmacists and some others engaged in pharmacy research, development, and teaching hold membership. This organization is a section of APhA.
7. *The American College of Apothecaries,* including some of the pharmacists who operate community pharmacies of the apothecary type. It is an affiliate of APhA.
8. *The National Pharmaceutical Association,* consisting of black pharmacists engaged in various aspects of pharmacy practice.
9. *The American Association of Colleges of Pharmacy,* in which all accredited colleges of pharmacy hold institutional membership. Faculty members and related associations may also hold membership.

In addition there are a number of newer groups representing a particular aspect of pharmacy or its practice such as the nursing home consultants and the radiopharmacy "specialists."

Beyond these voluntary associations there is the *National Association of Boards of Pharmacy,* to which the licensing bodies of the several states and jurisdictions belong. There is also the *American Council on Pharmaceutical Education,* the accrediting body for pharmacy educational institutions. In view of this multiplicity of organizations it is not surprising to find many diverse and divisive internal forces operating in the system of pharmacy.

The Study Commission believes that four sets of forces are of particular significance in predicting changes in the practice of pharmacy to be expected in the years to come. These are: (1) the direction of pharmaceutical research and development, (2) changes in pharmacy education, (3) attitudes and aspirations of pharmacists, and (4) the development of the concept of "clinical pharmacy." The balance of this chapter will be devoted to a brief discussion of these four forces.

Pharmaceutical Research and Development

The progress of science is most difficult to predict. No one knows with certainty when a major discovery will occur nor just what new knowledge can be developed into a safe, efficacious drug which will have a major impact upon therapy, prevention, or diagnosis of disease. However, from information about areas of current pharmaceutical research and from recognition of the factors which motivate and guide pharmaceutical research some informed guesses can be made. One thing is certain; there will be new, different, and more powerful drugs developed, produced, and marketed in the future. No one knows just what they will be, but there is reason to believe that some are more likely to appear than others.

The drive for success against communicable disease will continue, but will be primarily against viral diseases. In addition to better vaccines for influenza, there may be vaccines against hepatitis and against venereal diseases. There would appear to be also a chance of increasing the body's nonspecific resistance to various harmful factors.

Concerning the major challenges of cancer, heart disease, and mental illness, the great research thrust in neurobiology may lead to the identification of a biochemical basis for psychoses and a more effective chemotherapeutic treatment. The control of cancer will profit from the advances in immunology to provide vaccines effective against certain cancers and to give better surveillance for early detection. Against cardiovascular disease, tomorrow's pharmacologic solutions are most likely to be extensions of today's partial answers, the continuing battle against such predisposing factors as obesity, elevated blood pressure, abnormal blood lipids, and smoking. More effective and better tolerated antiarrhythmic drugs may be developed for chronic prophylactic administration to patients with coronary artery disease in order to prevent the enormous loss of life from sudden arrhythmias.

In medicine a shift in emphasis is already underway from the curing of episodes of illness to the maintenance of health, to concern with prevention and early detection of predisposition to disease. The effect of this on pharmacy will be that drugs used by healthy people are likely to be more numerous and more sophisticated. Such drugs as the tranquilizers and stimulants will be more specific in their actions. In the area of contraception, drugs will affect the mobility and implantation of the fertilized ovum by direct chemical actions with minimal other effects rather than by producing systemic hormonal changes. There will be drugs to increase intellectual acuity, to reduce obesity, and to minimize dependence on more harmful drugs including alcohol, tobacco, and other substances.

There are two important implications for the pharmacist in these futuristic speculations. First, he will have the familiar task of keeping up with the appearance of new and more sophisticated and more powerful chemotherapeutic agents. His chemical, biological, and pharmacological knowledge and understanding will need to be continually refurbished and expanded. Second, he will have to deal with a rapidly growing new category of drug products—so-called "drugs for healthy people." For most of history drugs have been developed, manufactured, prescribed, dispensed, and administered for the cure, amelioration, prevention, or diagnosis of disease. They have been associated with the presence or the threat of disease. The new class of drugs may be less associated with disease and more involved in assuring normal health. They are not consumed for therapeutic purposes but for a purpose defined by the consumer who desires to produce a result of value to him as an individual: the avoidance of pregnancy, the enhancement of intellectual acuity, the alteration of mood, even perhaps the mitigation of the aging process. One cannot predict whether these drugs will be dispensed only by prescription, or whether a third class of drugs will be created limited to sale on advice of a pharmacist, or whether they will be so safe that they will be available through over-the-counter sale. In any event the pharmacist will be dealing with new kinds of substances and with patients whose motivations do not arise as a reaction to illness, pain, or discomfort. Perhaps the users of these new drugs cannot be referred to as "patients" for they surely are not "sufferers" in the usual sense of this word. The participation of pharmacists in dispensing of oral contraceptives, the first of the "drugs for healthy people" to appear, has not been of major importance. These are prescription products but millions of units have been distributed by maternal health clinics without pharmacist participation. Thus, one must observe that pharmacists have not as yet demonstrated that their services will be essential to the proper dispensing and utilization of such products.

Pharmacy Education

Substantial changes have occurred in pharmacy education since the Elliott Report was published in 1950.[6] The recommendations of that report were not fully implemented. A curriculum of six years' duration beyond high school was recommended. Most colleges of pharmacy eventually decided upon a five-year course leading to a bachelor's degree. Two of the California colleges chose a six-year program leading to the degree of Doctor of Pharmacy. Graduate work has appeared in a number of colleges. These include the traditional PhD in the pharmaceutical sciences such as medicinal chemistry, and a professional degree called the Doctor of Pharmacy. It should be noted that this latter degree is currently acquired in several ways. On the one hand, some schools require one, two, or three years of additional study beyond the Bachelor of Pharmacy degree. On the other hand, it may be offered as an alternate to the bachelor's degree to students who are willing to devote additional time to obtaining a first professional degree.

The major change in pharmacy education has been greatly increased emphasis upon the basic physical, biological, and pharmaceutical sciences. These sciences have come to dominate the curriculum. The balance of the five years in the typical curriculum is devoted to general or liberal education and to the heterogeneous content referred to as "pharmacy administration." Recently instruction has been introduced described as "clinical pharmacy," but it clearly emphasizes services to *patients* who use drugs as contrasted to services connected only with drug *products*.

These changes of two decades in pharmacy education leave produced forces of change within pharmacy. In those years some 78,000 pharmacy students have been graduated and most of them have entered practice of some sort. It is inevitable that those graduates would wish to utilize the knowledge which they had gained and to practice skills they had developed. To the degree that their knowledge and skill were different from that of earlier graduates, and incongruent with the then current practice of pharmacy, and the pharmacy system, a certain amount of confrontation has occurred. Debate has been active within the profession and changes have resulted. Pharmacy education has clearly been one of the forces of change internal to pharmacy.

Attitudes, Motivations, and Aspirations of Pharmacists

Professions change in response to both external and internal forces, but response to such forces is greatly affected by the attitudes, motivations, and aspirations of the individual human beings who collectively comprise the profession. They may resist the forces of change, blunting them or changing their direction. They may welcome change and align themselves with the forces causing it.

One finds a great deal of dissatisfaction among some pharmacists; however, the nature of this feeling varies from group to group. Among independent community pharmacists one hears of resentment expressed in economic terms. It is stated that the independent community pharmacist receives smaller discounts on drug products purchased from manufacturers and wholesalers than do the drug chains. Thus, he must face difficult competition in prices for the prescription which he dispenses. Community pharmacists complain about the mountain of paperwork they must perform in order to obtain payment for services rendered to patients covered by Medicare, Medicaid, and other third-party payers and about long delays in receiving reimbursement. Staff pharmacists in both independent and chain community pharmacies complain that they spend their time in pouring, counting, and labeling—with little opportunity to use their full knowledge and professional skills.

Many pharmacists report difficulty in communicating with other health professionals, especially with physicians. They feel that pharmacy is treated as a peripheral profession, not in the mainstream of health services. Particularly among young pharmacists one finds resentment and discouragement that their practice has proven far less challenging in a professional sense than their education has prepared them for. One frequently hears the statement that the pharmacist is the most overeducated and the most underutilized of all professionals.

On the other hand, one finds pharmacists of all ages and in all settings who are satisfied, happy, and challenged by their practice. For the most part these individuals have taken the initiative to alter some of the aspects of their practice and to overcome some of the factors causing discontent and frustration. They have changed their practices in many different ways to improve their services, to find new ways to serve, to bring greater economic rewards, or to enter more directly into the mainstream of health care. This may be illustrated by the increasing number of pharmacists involved in hospitals or other institutional settings in recent years.

The motivations for change exhibited by pharmacists are as varied as their attitudes. Some are moved by a desire for greater economic rewards; some desire greater public recognition; some desire to be of greater service to patients and to the public in general. Whatever the motivation, one must report that the vast majority of pharmacists are motivated toward change. That change may be "back to the good old days" or "forward to a bright, although undefined, future." Most pharmacists are motivated toward change because most pharmacists are dissatisfied with the present for a variety of reasons.

Probably the greatest force is the desire of a growing number of pharmacists for a profession of greater service and stature. They wish to provide professional services of greater effectiveness to those they serve and to the public well-being. This has led to proposals for expanded roles and for new roles for pharmacists. Some of those proposed are highly controversial—such as the suggestion that the physician should diagnose the health problems of a patient and the pharmacist assume responsibility for drug therapy of the patient including the prescription of drugs. Other proposals suggest radical change in the places where pharmacists practice, such as moving the pharmacist from the drugstore to a consulting office. Another proposal is to place the hospital pharmacist at the patient's bedside administering medications, observing the progress of therapy, and altering it in accordance with his observations. One must report that there is a very positive force for change operating inside pharmacy—the desire and aspiration of a substantial number of pharmacists and pharmacy students who earnestly wish to provide more and better drug services to people who need those services.

The Movement to Clinical Pharmacy

Propelled by the motivations and aspirations of individual pharmacists and groups of pharmacists and by developments in pharmacy education, the past five to ten years have seen a growing movement toward a concept of "clinical pharmacy," as yet not clearly defined. In the past two years the developments in pharmacy education have been accelerated. The Congress, through the Health Manpower Act, has provided capitation grants to colleges of pharmacy with a mandate to incorporate instruction in "clinical pharmacy." There have been several attempts in organized pharmacy and in pharmacy education to provide a precise definition of the concept and of the term. As yet there is no unanimous agreement. The term "clinical pharmacy" was first used by a group of pharmacists engaged in developing drug information centers. Subsequently, it has been used to denominate a wide variety of practice roles developed by individual pharmacists, groups, and institutions of education and service. At the present it is possible therefore only to describe the area as a spectrum of individual, group, or institutional ideas. At the one end of the spectrum is the practice of an individual community pharmacist who has expanded his dispensing practices to include patient medication profiles, more frequent consultation with prescribing physicians and, particularly, improved communication with patients. The communication includes the reinforcement of the physician's instructions concerning administration, dosage, and timing; possible interactions with other drugs being used concurrently, with foods, or with alcohol; and expected therapeutic results. At the opposite end of the spectrum is the practice of a hospital pharmacist who is stationed in patient areas of the hospital participating regularly in prescribing decisions, monitoring patient response to therapy, taking drug histories and keeping detailed records of drug utilization and responses thereto, participating actively in the formulation of drug protocols and institutional drug policies, and providing drug information to physicians, nurses, and other health professionals. Such pharmacists can be described as integral members of the health care team providing direct patient care. In between these ends of the spectrum are many other forms of pharmacy practice including one or more of the needed services mentioned above. In a number of prepaid organized systems of health care, there are pharmacy services and pharmacy systems designed expressly to meet the needs of such organizations and their patients.

Although, as yet, there is no single definition of "clinical pharmacy" or of the knowledge, skills, and roles involved, it is clear that there is one common idea which is present in all of the manifestations; that idea is an emphasis upon *drugs* as they are *utilized* by and in the *patient.* It is the joining of *drug and patient* which is the inseparable and continuing concern of the evolving pharmacist. This is to be contrasted to the focus of the pharmacist only upon the drug *product,* its distribution, control, safekeeping, and dispensing. One must observe that although the concept of "clinical pharmacy" is still evolving, it should be regarded as a powerful force internal to pharmacy producing change in the system of pharmacy and in the practice of pharmacists. It is supported by the attitudes, motivations, and aspirations of a large number of individual pharmacists and by a growing emphasis in pharmacy education. It has further some public endorsement as represented by an action of the Congress, although we certainly are far away from the establishment of a public policy. At this time, the movement must be described as an internal factor for there is only little evidence that physicians, other health professionals, hospital administrators, or patients are urging that pharmacists provide clinical services. However, this situation may well change as other health professionals become more aware of the potential contributions to patient care.

The Study Commission is convinced that there are many and real gaps in the health care system as to knowledge, practices, procedures, organization, and communication which result in less than optimal benefit to patients who require drugs and drug therapy in order to recover or maintain health. The Commission is also convinced that properly educated and trained pharmacists can fill or, at least, narrow some of those gaps. The need is to identify precisely the gaps in which improved pharmacy services would be peculiarly effective in the improvement of patient care and the reduction of its cost. When that task is completed we shall have a rational definition of "clinical pharmacy." Eventually, perhaps that definition will describe the practice of the vast majority of pharmacists who should be deeply involved with people and their health needs as they are met through drugs.

IX. PHARMACISTS OF THE FUTURE

In the two preceding chapters, we have discussed forces both external and internal to pharmacy which are currently producing change and can be expected to produce further and accelerated change in the future. Some of these forces, particularly those producing change in the whole of the health care system, must be regarded as irresistible. Others involve some elements of choice to pharmacists in that they can choose to respond or not respond to opportunities to render new and expanded services. Thus, it is difficult to predict with certainty all of the roles pharmacists will play in the future and to detail exactly the knowledge and skills they must possess. However, it is the opinion of the Study Commission that there are substantial numbers of the pharmacy profession who are actively seeking ways to provide drug services of greater benefit to patients and society. It is reasonable to expect that in the future many pharmacists will choose to grasp these opportunities if they possess the required knowledge and skill to render them. Based upon these considerations, the Study Commission believes that some reasonably accurate predictions can be made concerning the pharmacists of the future.

It is virtually certain that the future will bring the greatest change in the lives of those pharmacists practicing in that portion of the system of pharmacy defined in Chapter II as dispensing. This is not to say that there will be no change in the practice of pharmacists in other parts of the system such as pharmaceutical research, manufacturing, and product distribution. However, change will be less in magnitude and will be less dramatic. Since by far the greatest number of pharmacists now practice, and in the future will practice, in the subsystem of drug dispensing, the changes of the future will affect the substantial majority of pharmacists.

Increasing organization and institutionalization will directly change the place where many pharmacists work. There is already a substantial growth in the number of hospital pharmacists. Although a smaller proportion of patients may be cared for in acute hospitals in the future, hospitals continue to grow in size. They will probably expand their outpatient services; they will add ambulatory clinics. Large group practices may initiate HMOs. Thus, the proportion of health services provided under the auspices of hospitals and their staffs will increase. Since drug therapy is involved in the treatment of most hospitalized patients and virtually all ambulatory patients, the necessity for a complete drug service on the premises will grow. More and more pharmacists will find practice opportunities in or under the auspices of hospitals, clinics, or other health service organizations.

The growing reliance upon pyschotropic drugs in the treatment of mental diseases is already making mental hospitals resemble more nearly other kinds of hospitals. As the modality of treatment becomes drug therapy, more and more pharmacists are required to dispense and administer medications, to maintain surveillance of drug utilization, to maintain drug and patient drug records, and to manage the drug delivery system. At the same time the length of patient stay in mental hospitals will continue to decrease. Many patients can be discharged when their illnesses are under reasonable control. They will receive continuing care under the supervision of a variety of health care personnel in community mental health centers. Since the primary means of disease control is one of continuing drug therapy, it follows that drug dispensing, utilization surveillance, patient drug records, patient counseling, and drug system management are required. All pharmacists providing such services will not necessarily be members of the staff of an institution but all will be members of an organization and will work within it. The significance of this observation is that there will be alternative modes of organization of health and medical services. One mode is institutional; another is a functional relationship between one or more community pharmacies and a community mental health center. Because not all pharmacy services will be provided in a single mode, it will be essential that there be regular and consistent communication between pharmacists practicing in the several modes so that continuity of optimal drug services to the patient can be maintained.

It must be expected that both the number and size of nursing homes will increase as the proportion of senior citizens in the total population grows. The growing numbers will demand more facilities for long-term care. Again, drug therapy is an important modality of care. More and more pharmacists will be involved in furnishing drug services in and to nursing homes. As some institutions grow in size they will provide full pharmacy services on their premises as do acute hospitals. Such institutions will require pharmacists to organize and manage their pharmacy systems, to maintain patient drug records, and to monitor drug utilization by patients. Smaller long-term care institutions will provide their pharmacy services using pharmacists as consultants or by contracting with community pharmacies.

Health maintenance organizations will continue to appear in many alternative forms. The proportion of health services furnished by such organizations will continue to increase. In many organizations pharmacy services will be furnished on the premises. In others they will be furnished through organized plans involving community pharmacies and pharmacists.

One must conclude that in the future we shall see an increasing proportion of dispensing pharmacists working in institutions providing acute, chronic, and/or ambulatory care. Increasing numbers of pharmacists will also be working within organized plans although the place of work may still be in various types of community pharmacies.

Change in the degree of organization of pharmacy practice will involve a corresponding change in the nature of relationships. The dispensing pharmacist shifts from being a solo practitioner to being a member of a group furnishing a comprehensive health service of which drug services are an integral part. Such a change demands capacities of collaboration with other pharmacists and other health professionals. Decisions are made cooperatively rather than individually. Drug records become a part of total patient records. The procurement, storage, care, and dispensing of drugs must be organized as a system. The community pharmacy as we know it today will become a subsystem of an integrated health service rather than a self-contained enterprise devoted exclusively to dispensing drugs. Another facet of institutionalization and organization is a change in relation to other health workers. The present relationship of pharmacist to physician in community pharmacy is best described as intermittent and at arm's length. In an organization in which pharmacist and physician are both employees the relationship may become constant and is face to face. Similar relationships can develop between pharmacists and nurses and other health professionals. Even in a noninstitutionalized organization, interprofessional relations under planned and systematic arrangements are necessary. As systems become larger and more complex further division of labor inevitably occurs. The differentiation of those with managerial responsibilities increases. Efficiency requires the assignment of some tasks to less highly trained workers; the work of such aides requires systematic supervision. Again, interpersonal skills and habits are required as a fundamental attribute.

The relationship to patients will change for many dispensing pharmacists under growing organization and institutionalization. As a member of a health service organization the pharmacist will be responsible for more than the delivery of a product to the ultimate consumer. It is certain that he will be responsible for reinforcing the physician's instructions about drug therapies. He will be responsible for keeping patient utilization records. This will necessitate that he elicit information from the patient concerning his total use of drugs, his compliance with instructions, his reports of effects, reactions, and interactions. Further, with the growth of prepaid plans the pharmacist will see patients much more regularly than is currently the case. A more personal and continuing relationship with the patient should develop. The pharmacist will dispense drugs, and he will both dispense and elicit information concerning drug usage and concerning the patient.

Institutionalization and other forms of organization have involved changes in the mode of compensating pharmacists for their services. Institutional pharmacists are very generally salaried employees. Pharmacists involved in other forms of organization, such as HMOs, are frequently salaried. Other pharmacists are compensated under contractual arrangements involving retainers, dispensing fees or capitation payments. In all cases we see a shift from the familiar form of paying the pharmacist in connection with the number of drug products which he dispenses to paying the pharmacist for his total drug services which may or may not involve the physical delivery of a drug product. The essential difference is compensation for *knowledge and skill,* used to meet individual or social needs rather than for just handling the product.

Regulation of the pharmacist's activities will increase in the future. It is certain that professional standards review mechanisms will involve drug utilization as a central aspect of health care. The pharmacist will be required to maintain both patient and institutional records and to monitor both patient and institutional drug utilization. Such records will also include cost data to make possible cost/benefit reviews. By the nature of organizations there must be protocols for the operation of an institution and the definition of the responsibilities and practice of each health worker in the organization. Thus, both through external requirements and internal demands the pharmacist will find his practice increasingly standardized and regulated.

All of the changes in pharmacy practice which have been discussed above have implications for the knowledge and skills required of the dispensing pharmacist of the future. In the past the requisite knowledge and skill have dealt with the several aspects of handling and dispensing a drug product. The knowledge involved has been chemical and pharmacological. The skill has been essentially mechanical and related to a physical material, its acquisition, protection, control, and distribution. In the future the knowledge and skill must be of drugs *and of people.* The essence of dispensing is the interface between a chemical material and a patient. Knowledge about the substance *and about the person* who is to consume the substance is essential. The action of a drug upon the patient depends upon his physiology and other biological functions, upon the status of his health or his illness, upon his social, cultural, and emotional nature. If the pharmacist is to be responsible for facilitating and monitoring drug therapy of a patient he must possess knowledge about that patient as a biological, social, cultural, and emotional being. The knowledge required of the pharmacist of the future must encompass not only the physical and biological sciences but also the behavioral and social sciences as well. The skills required of the future pharmacist must be those of dealing with a drug as a biologically active chemical and those of dealing with the complexities of a living and behaving human individual. These are skills of observation and communication, of data gathering, recording, and interpretation; these are skills of synthesis and judgment; these are skills of interpersonal relations, of management, and of collaboration and cooperation.

The future will certainly bring increased emphasis in two areas of health service—primary care and preventive medicine. There are several forces at work which demand such increased emphasis—societal need, public expectations and the necessity to control the rapidly escalating costs of health services. Means must and will be found to care for the episodes of self-limiting disease and minor injuries in effective and economical ways. It is obviously more effective and cheaper to prevent disease and disability than to care for illness. In addition to the proliferation of ambulatory clinics and other forms of HMOs we must expect the development of large efforts aimed at preventing obesity, alcoholism and other types of drug abuse, and destructive lifestyles which predispose to illness, disease, disability, and untimely death.

An important part of primary care and a large part of preventive medicine is self-care. In turn, self-care is dependent upon the information given to and understood by the individual patient. We must look forward to the development of programs to educate and inform our citizens about matters of health so that they may make more informed and more rational decisions which will improve and maintain their health. Such information must deal with diet, with lifestyle, with the effect of environment, and with the use of drugs. Self-selection and administration of drugs is a prominent part of self-care.

Pharmacists will be expected to play important roles both in improving primary care and in preventive medicine. Since drugs play so prominent a part in both areas, drug information and understanding are of central importance. Pharmacists are a part of physician-directed primary care and preventive medicine and of self-care as well. It is the pharmacist who knows something about a patient's habits with reference to OTC drugs and has perhaps the best chance to advise him concerning them. If pharmacists are to participate actively in primary and preventive care, it will not be so much as dispensers of drugs but rather as *dispensers of drug information* both to the individual and to the community. The skills required are those of communication and education; the knowledge required is that of drugs and their actions and of human behavior.

The future will produce less change in the practice of a pharmacist engaged in the several pharmacy roles in the drug industry. The activity of research and development will change little although the knowledge will be more complex and involve therefore more specialization and perhaps some new scientific disciplines. Furthermore, the demand for a freer flow of knowledge and information about drugs will require additional knowledge and communicative skill on the part of those pharmacists involved in drug distribution.

The area of drug information will become increasingly significant. As there is more knowledge, as physicians demand more information about drugs, as dispensing pharmacists require more information, as patients require both drug products and information about them, a more complete information system must develop. More pharmacists practicing in drug information systems will be required. The information system will have to be more complex, more complete, more responsive, and more efficient. This will involve the use of sophisticated information technology, the use of computers, and effective communication systems.

Several times in this report, the Study Commission has described pharmacy as a differentiated system. In this system pharmacists perform specific roles within one of the steps or subsystems. There is no such thing as "the pharmacist." One must always speak in the plural for there are many roles to be played and no individual plays all of them. The forces of change described above predict even greater differentiation in the future. There will continue to be the differentiation between research, development, manufacturing, distribution, and dispensing; there will also be differentiation between those involved in acute, chronic, and ambulatory care; there will be differentiation between those who work in institutions and those who work in less formal organizations; there will be differentiation between those who work as managers of systems and those who work directly with patients.

To many observers the basic differentiations already established and the further differentiations to be expected indicate that there may be a great deal of specialization in pharmacy in the future. Already there is discussion of formal recognition of specialization with the organization of specialty boards and specialty certification. To the Study Commission such an outcome may not be wholly in the best interest of the pharmacy profession. The profession is already fractionated into multiple special interest groups. If each group is to be further partitioned into specialties the profession will soon become a set of independent and isolated groups, each concerned with a little part of the whole. Few will be concerned with the whole and there will be no one to speak for pharmacy as an integrated, logical, and essential knowledge system or to encourage its rational evolution.

Some will argue that differentiation and specialization are synonymous—that since pharmacists are differentiated they are automatically specialized. In the judgment of the Study Commission the two words are not synonymous. Differentiation occurs because of differences in place of practice (e.g., in a community pharmacy versus a hospital); because of differences in function (e.g., systems management versus patient service); because of differences in patients served (e.g., acutely ill versus chronically ill), and because of differences in compensation arrangements (e.g., prepaid plans versus fee-for-service). Specialization occurs because of uniqueness of service not because of uniqueness of place, of function, or patient service. We can conceive of the radiopharmacist as a specialist. He must have unique pharmacy knowledge—pharmacy knowledge that other pharmacists do not have and do not need. On the other hard, we do not view hospital pharmacy as a specialty. There is no strictly pharmacy knowledge which is unique to such practice that is not possessed by many pharmacists working in other settings. We cannot view those who furnish consultative services to nursing homes as specialists. Again, there is no unique body of pharmacy knowledge nor unique pharmacy skill which is not also essential for pharmacy services in other environments of patient care.

The Study Commission makes these observations for several reasons. The specialization and superspecialization which has occurred in the medical profession has brought many benefits to patients but has also created some serious problems. Medicine has become fractionated. Medical care has become discontinuous, episodic, and anything but comprehensive. Now we as a nation are engaged in attempts to compensate for these shortcomings; we are trying to encourage the education of more primary physicians; we are encouraging more organization of health care services so that patients may expect greater continuity and comprehensiveness of care. There are probably lessons to be learned by pharmacy from the example of medicine. Specialization does increase costs to the professional and thus to the patient. Costs incurred anywhere in the system must be paid for and the only source of payment is the person who receives its services, namely, the *patient.* In this time of great concern about the costs of health services, it would seem unwise to take any steps that involve additional costs without assurance of tangible and valuable increments in the quality and effectiveness of patient care. Finally, the Study Commission reiterates the observation that pharmacy is already a divided profession. What is needed is more unity, not more divisiveness. Thus, we urge the most serious consideration of any proposal to form a large number of specialties and their attendant paraphernalia. The ultimate question to be answered is how can the profession be ordered so that our ultimate concern, *the patient,* be best served—not how can the individual pharmacist be set apart from his professional comrades?

X. THE OBJECTIVES OF PHARMACY EDUCATION AND THE RESPONSIBILITIES OF SCHOOLS OF PHARMACY

The Study Commission advances the following generalized and inclusive statement of the objectives of pharmacy education.

The overall objectives of pharmacy education are to prepare persons with a ready knowledge of all aspects of drugs, their actions upon and uses by patients, so that graduates may possess competencies to serve individual and societal drug needs.

We call attention to three key elements in this definition: first, ready and comprehensive knowledge of drugs, their actions and use; second, competencies to serve; third, service to meet both individual and societal needs.

Pharmacy is today, and will be in the future, a differentiated profession. By no means are all pharmacists alike, nor are their funds of knowledge identical nor their professional skills the same, nor their environments of practice shared by all. The differentiation of pharmacists and their practices fall into three general categories. First, there is minimal differentiation without appreciable difference in pharmacy knowledge and skill. Examples of this category would be the difference in practice between a staff pharmacist in an independent community pharmacy and one in a chain pharmacy; the difference between a community pharmacist's practice and that of a staff pharmacist in an ambulatory health care center; the difference between the practice of a staff pharmacist in a general hospital and that of a staff pharmacist in a large nursing home. Second, there is differentiation with substantial difference in the *character* of total professional knowledge and skill. Examples of this category would be the difference between the practice of a staff pharmacist in a large acute hospital and that of community pharmacist; the difference between the practice of a radiopharmacist and a drug information specialist; the difference between a pharmacist engaged in industrial research and development and a pharmacist directing the pharmacy services system of a large and complex HMO. Third, there is differentiation with significant difference in the *amount, complexity, and sophistication* of total professional knowledge and its constituent skills. Examples of substantial differentiated roles are pharmaceutical research, management of complex systems, and university teaching.

It is the opinion of the Study Commission that in spite of the real and multifaceted differentiation in the practice roles of pharmacists, there is a common body of knowledge, skill, attitudes, and behavior which all pharmacists must possess. In a practical and detailed sense the objectives of pharmacy education must be stated in terms of both the common knowledge and skill and of the differentiated and/or additional knowledge and skill required for specific practice roles. This can be done only by stating a series of limited educational objectives, which if met in sequential order will accomplish both common and differentiated objectives. Further, the objectives must be accomplished within reasonable time limitations and within the strictures of prudent use of educational resources and the reality of effective use of financial means.

The Study Commission offers the following statement of the minimum objectives of the first professional degree in pharmacy, i.e., the first level of the limited objectives of pharmacy education.

1. The inculcation of the knowledge, attitudes, and habits which are common to the practice of pharmacy in all of its differentiated roles.
2. The translation of that knowledge into the skills common to pharmacy practice in the several roles which are not differentiated by additional knowledge and practice experience.
3. The development of a familiarity with the nature and requirements of the practice roles which do require additional knowledge and more complex skills to orient students to the career options open to them.

The successful meeting of these first objectives would equip the graduate for entry into practice at an initial level in several alternative roles and provide him with the understanding necessary for intelligent decisions concerning further education and/or training.

The second of the limited objectives of pharmacy education to be considered are the competencies to perform those differentiated practice roles which require additional knowledge and skill. Clearly such learning ought to follow the attainment of that knowledge and skill described as the minimum to be accomplished within the first professional degree and be closely articulated to it. Further, it is obvious that the amount and character of additional learning required for competence in such differentiated roles varies quite widely from role to role; thus, to achieve the appropriate competence for any specific differentiated role requires an educational program specifically tailored to the needs of that role. In some instances what is needed is a substantial amount of practice in that role and only a modest amount of formally acquired additional knowledge. It would seem that an educational model akin to the residency in medicine would be appropriate. In such a case the program should be the joint responsibility of a college of pharmacy and the service institution in which the experience takes place. Such a program may or may not result in an advanced degree at the option of the educational institution. In any case the educational institution must take full responsibility for the quality of instruction wherever it is given. The model suggested would seem appropriate for the differentiated pharmacy roles in hospital pharmacies, chronic care institutions, or HMOs. For other differentiated roles such as drug information pharmacist some additional practice would be required but also large amounts of didactic instruction in information theory and technology and in communication. Such an educational program would have to be the responsibility of an educational institution and in all probability should lead to an advanced professional degree.

It should be noted that at this point the Study Commission has proposed objectives in two steps—a basic minimum for a first degree to produce an undifferentiated pharmacist and a subsequent education or training of flexibility directed to differentiation with competence. Traditionally, the first professional degree has been a baccalaureate. The Commission foresees that as the responsibilities of pharmacists approach those described in Chapter IX, the minimum objectives of the first professional degree in pharmacy will need to embrace an enlarging or changing core of knowledge and skills. Further, it is proposed that additional knowledge and experiences in one or more of the differentiated roles will become an essential component of preparation for practice.

Whatever may be the title finally selected for the first professional degree, the Commission believes the future responsibilities of pharmacists described in Chapter IX will require an alteration of the range of knowledge and skills expected of its graduates. The Commission urges schools of pharmacy to experiment with curricular modifications intended to include the necessary core of knowledge and experiences to prepare for these responsibilities. Since such a program would involve a more extensive and diverse curriculum and greater performance expectations of its graduates than is currently the case with the baccalaureate program, it may warrant in the judgment of the granting institution, a degree higher than the baccalaureate.

While this first professional degree program should develop to include preparation for some differentiated roles in pharmacy, it cannot be expected to equip each of its graduates for entry into all possible roles in pharmacy. It will be necessary for those who wish to fulfill more highly differentiated roles to continue their education beyond the first professional degree. Recognition of such advanced educational experiences may be through further degree designations or certifications.

The third limited objective of pharmacy education deals with those differentiated roles which require much additional knowledge and, of equal importance, knowledge of much greater complexity and sophistication. Further, substantially different and additional skills are needed. Proper preparation for such pharmacy roles may be, as appropriate in the individual case, through graduate or advanced professional degrees. A pharmacist who aspires to a role in research in biochemistry needs an advanced degree in biochemistry, e.g., an MS or PhD. A pharmacist who aspires to the role of manager of a complex drug system may need an advanced degree in management, e.g., an MBA. The pharmacist who aspires to a career in drug regulation may need a degree in law, e.g., a JD. Some of the required educational opportunities may be within the competence of the colleges of pharmacy, e.g., PhD in medicinal chemistry or pharmacokinetics. Additional opportunities already exist in other departments, e.g., a PhD in biochemistry, in management science, information theory, or in public health. Thus, in describing this portion of pharmacy education, we must deal not only with the school of pharmacy but with the whole of the university.

Responsibilities of the College of Pharmacy

The primary and overriding responsibility of a college of pharmacy is to its students. It is responsible for furnishing the minds of its students with the requisite knowledge, equipping their minds and hands with the necessary skills, molding their habits, and encouraging those attitudes and motivations which are essential to successful, effective, and satisfying practice in one of the many roles of pharmacy. The content, the environment, and the process of the appropriate learning experience will be discussed in detail in Chapters XI and XII. Beyond this primary responsibility to its students, the school of pharmacy has responsibilities to its faculty, to the pharmacy profession, to the pharmaceutical industry, to the public, and, if they should develop, to pharmacy technicians.

The Faculty

The excellence or lack of excellence of any educational experience depends directly upon the quality of the members of the faculty, their scholarship, their teaching proficiency, their motivation, and their ability to serve as role models in the practice of pharmacy. Hence, the school of pharmacy must provide its faculty members with opportunities for mature learning so that they may become and remain scholars; with opportunities to acquire proficiency as teachers; with opportunities to develop high standards of competence as practitioners.

The matter of faculty research needs comment. Research should be conceived as a means to three quite separate and distinct ends. First, it is the means by which mature students, which faculty members surely should be, continue their own self-directed learning. Thus, they become and remain scholars. Second, research is the means by which new knowledge is generated. Third, it is the means by which real and practical problems are solved. Pharmacy aspires to be a learned profession. Therefore, its educational leaders must be learned. To be learned they must have the opportunity to become and to remain scholars. This they can do only if they have opportunities for self-directed and continued learning. The greatest proportion of new knowledge about drugs is generated in the research laboratories of the drug industry. This is in sharp contrast to other health sciences. In the medical schools the faculties generate the bulk of scientific research and the new knowledge which contributes to the advancement of medical practice. There are many important problems in the practice of pharmacy and questions about drugs particularly in biopharmaceutics and pharmacokinetics which are and remain problems because of lack of knowledge. They need to be identified and studied. This suggests that faculty research in schools of pharmacy should be concentrated upon problems of *pharmacy practice* and upon the gaps in drug knowledge. The benefit to faculty scholarship would be the same, but in addition real and practical problems would be solved, and the effectiveness of pharmacy education greatly enhanced.

The matter of practice opportunities for members of pharmacy school faculties is also of importance. The objective of pharmacy education is to prepare students to *practice*. It is not sufficient to educate them only to know; they must also be trained to do. This requires that some of their teachers be actively engaged in doing, that is engaged in the exemplary practice of pharmacy. No one would be satisfied with a medical faculty which did not have a substantial number of its members caring for patients. Students learn by precept and by example, probably more by the latter. They seek role models and emulate them. We realize that it is not easy to provide faculty practice opportunities. However, they are absolutely necessary. The Study Commission strongly recommends that every college of pharmacy promptly find the ways and means to provide appropriate practice opportunities for its faculty members having clinical teaching responsibilities.

The Profession

The schools of pharmacy have several responsibilities to the profession of pharmacy. The most obvious is to educate and train those who are to become members of the profession in the future; but the responsibility does not end with graduation of the student. New knowledge is generated, new drugs and technologies are developed, new demands and expectations for drug services arise from society and from individual patients. The professional pharmacist must therefore be a continuing learner. A well-organized and accessible system of continuing education is required. The responsibility for organizing and maintaining such a system must be borne jointly by the professional organizations of pharmacy and the colleges of pharmacy. The colleges, being the locus of educational expertise, must respond to the need of the profession and provide both the knowledge and pedagogical expertise required.

A second responsibility to the profession is the dissemination of new knowledge and technology. As the colleges of pharmacy direct their research efforts to the solution of problems of practice, there will be knowledge to be shared promptly with the practicing profession. It may be that the usual channels of communication, such as professional journals, will not be the most effective way of communicating to the total profession. Seminars, workshops, short courses may be found more effective. Television, video tapes, and other learning aids can be helpful.

Pharmacy has one continuing problem—that is the flow of drug information. Some colleges of pharmacy have interested themselves in the matter and have established and maintained drug information centers. Most observers agree that these centers have not been widely used and have proved rather costly. Clearly much research and study are required to determine how drug information can be made readily and economically available to the practicing pharmacist, to the physician, the nurse, the patient, and the public. This is one of the real and practical problems crying for research in colleges of pharmacy.

The Pharmaceutical Industry

The colleges of pharmacy have responsibilities to the pharmaceutical industry and the industry has responsibilities to the colleges. A significant number of the graduates of colleges of pharmacy find their roles of practice in the industry—in research, in development, in manufacturing, and in distribution. The colleges have the responsibility of knowing in detail the knowledge and skills which are required by pharmacists in their several industrial roles. This, in turn, requires a continuing communication and relationship between pharmacy education and the industry. Some observers have remarked upon the isolation of pharmacy education. Few, if any, colleges have established functioning relationships with the pharmaceutical industry. This isolation is particularly unfortunate with reference to the flow of information about new drug products and the flow of other pharmacy information. The colleges do not develop the bulk of new drug knowledge; the pharmaceutical companies do. If future pharmacists are to be furnished with the most recent knowledge there must be a system of communication between pharmacy education and the industry and the industry should provide learning opportunities for students.

The Public

The Study Commission in this Report has observed frequently that the system of pharmacy is highly effective in supplying drug products to the public, but quite ineffective in supplying necessary drug information to those who actually utilize those products, namely, *patients*. There is need for widespread education concerning drugs and their use. The colleges of pharmacy do have a public responsibility to provide an adequate number of well-educated and trained pharmacists who will establish relationships with individual patients; but this is not the only responsibility. Students must be trained and motivated to teach patients about drugs and to evaluate the efficacy of such teaching. Beyond this, the general public has the right to be more fully informed about drugs. With their expertise the colleges of pharmacy surely have a responsibility to participate in the broad dissemination of information to the public. Relationships to schools, to consumer groups, and to the mass media need to be established and maintained.

The Pharmacy Technician

The questions about pharmacy technicians continue to be hotly debated. In many states their utilization is technically illegal. Yet there are aides of various kinds being used in community pharmacies, in hospitals, and in ambulatory care clinics. It is the opinion of the Study Commission that the utilization of technicians will increase as more and more health services are delivered under organized and institutionalized auspices. The characteristic of organizations is the division of labor. Physicians' assistants and nurses' aides are employed. It seems highly probable that pharmacists' aides will also be employed in ever increasing numbers.

When this occurs, pharmacy technicians will become a recognized part of the system of drug dispensing. As their duties and roles become defined the question as to their proper training will have to be answered. The definition of that training will be the joint responsibility of the pharmacy profession, pharmacy education, and the state boards of pharmacy. The general supervision of the training, however, should be the responsibility of the colleges of pharmacy. The role of the pharmacy technician can be rationally defined only in terms of the pharmacist's role. The education of the pharmacy technician can be defined rationally only in terms of the pharmacist's education. This is not to say that the colleges of pharmacy must be ready to undertake the sole responsibility for actual education and training of technicians. Other kinds of institutions, such as community colleges and health care institutions, can participate collaboratively in the education of technicians. However, the pharmacy colleges must play a significant and active role in the curriculum design, in the setting of standards, and in supervising the teaching of pharmacy technicians. Further, if pharmacists are to utilize and supervise technicians, such workers must be present both as students and workers in the clinical setting in which pharmacists learn their skills of practice. No one would think of educating a graduate nurse who was to work with nurses' aides or nursing technicians in a hospital in which none of the latter were employed. If pharmacists are to use technicians the learning to work with them must be a part of professional education. Further continuing education will be particularly needed for pharmacy technicians. Such programs must be coordinated with those for professional pharmacists since the knowledge and skills of both must be advanced simultaneously. The pharmacy educational system must assume a major responsibility for all programs of continuing education.

XI. THE CONTENT OF PHARMACY EDUCATION

It is comparatively easy to develop a statement of the broad objectives of an educational program. It is much more difficult to describe the details of a program which can accomplish the objectives. It is not the function of the Study Commission on Pharmacy to recommend the ideal curriculum which will ensure the proper education of the pharmacist of the future. The competence and the responsibility for this demanding task lie with the faculties of the colleges of pharmacy. It is they who must implement chosen programs; it is they who must justify them to students and to society. The colleges of pharmacy collectively have a powerful tool to assist them in the American Association of Colleges of Pharmacy. Happily, the Association is already deeply involved in studying the important questions of curricular content and of educational process. The individual colleges should participate actively in the debate and make full use of the collective findings. However, the Study Commission wishes to make some observations about the content of pharmacy education in relation to the objectives it has proposed. The preparation of every professional must include by definition both knowledge and skill. Professionals are people who know and who use their knowledge to do. We present our thoughts on content under two categories—knowledge and skill.

Knowledge

The choice of curricular content begins with the question of relevance. Because drugs are chemical substances which produce biological effects, it is evident that chemical and biological knowledge is relevant to pharmacy. But chemistry has a number of branches: inorganic, organic, physical, analytical, synthetic, natural products. Biology has several branches: physiology, anatomy, pathology, to name but three. In addition there are hybrid disciplines which combine both chemical and biological knowledge: biochemistry, pharmacology, biophysics, pharmacokinetics. Because drugs are utilized by human individuals who are biological organisms and complex persons shaped by psychological, emotional, cultural, and economic forces, it is evident that psychological, social, and economic knowledge is also relevant to pharmacy. Since drugs are developed, manufactured, distributed, and dispensed in a system and systems have to be operated and managed, it is evident that the managerial sciences—organization science, economics, computer science, information science—are relevant to pharmacy. From these intuitive answers to the questions of relevance, one can draw up a list of sciences (knowledge) which must be included in the education of the pharmacist.

At this point those responsible for the pharmacy curriculum are faced with the vexing questions of what and of how much of each science shall be included within a curriculum given the fact that there must be a rational limit on the time devoted by a student to a course of professional study. One approach is the attempt to broaden, cover the essentials of each of the sciences in as short a time as possible. This might be called a curriculum determined by the amount of knowledge available in each of the relevant disciplines. An alternative approach is to start with the question of what it is that the pharmacist must be able to *do well.* If these functions can be defined clearly, the knowledge needed to perform them with confidence can be identified. This approach can be called designing a curriculum in accordance with desired competencies. In the opinion of the Study Commission this is by far the most desirable course of action.

We must recognize that pharmacy education is in a most difficult situation. Many roles or tasks have been suggested for pharmacists but they have not been scientifically analyzed as to the competencies involved. It is difficult, if not impossible, to identify with precision the relevant science basic to a competency which has not been clearly defined and evaluated. Other health professions have faced this dilemma and have found only one way to solve it. In the case of medical education it required the development within the medical faculty a cadre of a particular kind of hybrid scholar—the clinical scientist. A clinical scientist in medicine is one who is equally at home and equally expert as a physician at the patient's bedside and as a basic scientist in the laboratory. It is he who is best able to discern the exact portion of his science which is specifically and peculiarly relevant to the care he must give to his patient with a particular disease condition. He, therefore, is able to assist his colleagues in making the choice of those parts of his scientific discipline which must be given the highest priority within the curriculum.

Pharmacy faculties have a substantial number of well-trained basic scientists in chemistry, medicinal chemistry, pharmacology, and pharmaceutics. They have some truly competent behavioral and social scientists. Some faculties have highly competent pharmacy practitioners, the counterpart of clinical physicians. However, pharmacy faculties have very few members who can be called clinical scientists—people who are equally skilled and trained in a science and in pharmacy practice. It is probably correct to point out that there is a handful of such people, namely, the clinical pharmacokineticists who actually serve patients by the measurement of drug levels in the blood in order to improve therapy in complex disease situations. There are a few other individuals in the pharmacy system who might also be called clinical scientists. The pharmacist in industry responsible for dosage formulation is practicing one of the roles of pharmacy and must also be a scientist in medicinal chemistry and pharmaceutics. Still pharmacy education does suffer from a lack of an adequate number and variety of clinical scientists and there is, therefore, an inadequate link between the knowledge of pharmacy and the art of pharmacy practice. This presents a most difficult problem to the faculties as they endeavor to plan a rational curriculum based on clearly defined competencies needed for a truly professional practice.

In the view of the Study Commission the greatest contribution which a foundation or governmental agency could make to upgrade pharmacy education, and thereby improve drug services to the public, would be to fund a national program to train a modest number of clinical scientists for pharmacy. One can envision a program to give a hundred or more well-trained pharmacy practitioners the opportunity to acquire deeper scientific knowledge, the skill of rigorous research, and broadened understanding of the management and control of disease. As such persons completed their advanced training they should find important places on pharmacy faculties and fill the void which is so evident.

However, even if such a fortunate event should occur, it would be a number of years before such individuals would be available and would have the opportunity to furnish their badly needed services to pharmacy education. The colleges of pharmacy need to begin now on the improvement of their educational programs. There is an alternative to the suggested program of training a cadre of clinical scientists which can be implemented immediately and could be substantially helpful. The clinical members of the pharmacy faculties could undertake careful and scientific study of the unmet needs of patients, physicians, nurses, and institutions in the area of drug services, devise experimental programs to meet one or more of those unmet needs, and keep precise records of their operation, outcomes, benefits, and costs. The continuing review of such programs jointly by the practitioners and the basic scientists of the faculty would lead to a more precise definition of the competencies required and the identification of the relevant knowledge. The continuing association of scientists and practitioners in devising, operating, and measuring well-planned experimental programs would provide the link between knowledge and skill which the clinical scientist provides because of his dual education and interest. It is the opinion of the Study Commission that one or both of these suggestions must be implemented before pharmacy education can reach a satisfactory level of quality or practicality.

There are some general observations which the Study Commission wishes to make concerning the knowledge content of pharmacy education. The present curriculum seems to be out of balance. Knowledge about drugs appears to be much more heavily stressed than knowledge about people. An inspection of the catalogue of almost any college of pharmacy reveals that departments of chemistry, medicinal chemistry, pharmacology, and pharmaceutics have sizable rosters. The course offerings in physical and biological science are numerous and extensive. In sharp contrast there are no departments of behavioral, social, economic, and managerial sciences. Frequently there is only a department called "pharmacy administration"—a traditional term which originally had a narrow connotation but has now broadened to be a catchall for behavioral and social sciences. The course offerings in the sciences other than physical and biological are few in number and frequently of limited extent even in universities with a full offering in those disciplines. One must conclude that the present-day pharmacy graduates have much greater knowledge of drug products and their effects on the human organism than they have of human behavior, cultural determinants, health service systems and their economics. Clearly pharmacists must have ready knowledge about drugs, but they also must have ready knowledge about people, about relationships and communication with them, and about systems and costs of service. The Study Commission reiterates the point that pharmacy is a knowledge system in which chemical substances and people called *patients* meet and interact. Needed and optimally effective drug therapy results only when both drugs and those who consume them are fully understood. We suggest that one of the first steps in reviewing the educational program of a college of pharmacy should be the weighing of the relative emphasis given to the physical and biological sciences as against the behavioral and social sciences.

Pharmacy Skills

The consideration of the skills (competencies) both generic and differentiated needed for effective pharmacy practice requires a different approach from that taken in thinking about knowledge. With knowledge the overriding consideration is relevance. With skills the overriding consideration is with need, effectiveness, and cost. In its several meetings, the Study Commission has received testimony from many and diverse sources. The testimony has been in response to these questions: What do pharmacists do? What can pharmacists do? What should pharmacists do? There appears to be a consensus in the answers to the first question. Pharmacists deal effectively and competently with drug products, their manufacture, their distribution, their dispensing. The answers to the second question were more varied but did have a remarkable agreement as to what pharmacists *cannot* now do well. The most frequently mentioned were lack of skill in communication with patients and physicians or nurses, lack of skill in management, and lack of skill in recording and using drug information about patients—their utilization of and reaction to drugs. Responses to the third question were even more varied. Opinions were expressed that pharmacists should do many of the things they do not now do—they should communicate with patients and with other health professionals, devise and operate more effective and economical systems of drug delivery, keep more complete and meaningful patient drug records, assist in education of the public concerning drugs and drug usage. All of the items in this list are unmet needs. Because they involve drugs and people they are unmet needs of the pharmacy system, and, intuitively, should and can be met by pharmacists. But there is not at this time a precise definition of how they are to be met nor of the competencies required to meet them. There is little measurement of their benefits nor of their costs. The Study Commission reiterates its opinion that data must be obtained by some means about benefits and about costs. Only then can a rational answer be given to the question of what pharmacists should do; only then can pharmacy education determine the skills which must be inculcated and competencies developed.

There are three generic intellectual skills requisite to practice of any health service profession. These are the skills of problem identification and of problem solving and the skills and habits of continuing learning. These skills are developed as the product of specific learning experiences and of the total impact of an extended learning program. They are both skills and habits, both competencies and attitudes. Further, they involve a continuing motivation. As the list of desired skills is developed for a competency determined curriculum these three generic intellectual skills must be included.

XII. THE ENVIRONMENT OF PHARMACY EDUCATION

The effect upon the student of any educational program is largely determined by the appropriateness of the curriculum, the vitality of the teaching, and the quality of the educational environment. If the education of future pharmacists is to achieve greater effectiveness and higher quality, we must be concerned with curriculum, teachers, and educational environment. The environment can and does limit a curriculum. It may be impossible to develop a sound curriculum in a limited environment because needed instruction, physical facilities, or practice opportunities are not available.

Because pharmacy is a profession, pharmacy education demands a learning experience in which both knowledge and skill can be mastered. Because pharmacy is a health profession, pharmacy education demands an environment in which the sciences relevant to the practice of a health service are available. Because pharmacists must practice in association with other health workers, pharmacy education demands an environment in which other health professionals are being educated and other health professions are being practiced. Thus, the ideal environment for pharmacy education will be an institution of university level possessing teaching resources in the full range of the sciences—physical, biological, behavioral, social, economic, and managerial—engaged in instruction for the health professions, and responsible for the delivery of health services to patients. There is only one educational environment which could fulfill all of these criteria, namely, the complete university health science center. Further, the active participation of well-trained pharmacist practitioner-teachers would improve the education of other professionals such as physicians and nurses. However, it must be observed that a number of university health science centers fall short of being ideal environments. They may have fine resources in all the disciplines; they may be engaged in educating a variety of health professionals; they may have access to many clinical teaching facilities. Yet, students of pharmacy, medicine, and nursing do not learn together. Physicians, nurses, pharmacists do not practice together. The needed elements are present but for various reasons, most of which are human in character, they do not produce the performance nor the atmosphere essential to a constructive environment. Above all, physicians, dentists, nurses must recognize that the full discharge of their responsibilities would be improved by well-educated pharmacists and that they should contribute to the education of pharmacy students and will benefit from the information and education pharmacists may provide.

It is the opinion of the Study Commission that even if all university health science centers were functioning as the ideal learning environment, it would still be impractical to recommend that all colleges of pharmacy be relocated immediately in university health science centers. The Commission believes that the substantial *majority* of colleges of pharmacy should be so located for only there can the full range of knowledge, skill, and practice be found. However, not all colleges of pharmacy are parts of universities and not all universities have health science centers. Further, the number of centers which are prepared to participate in pharmacy education is limited. To limit the number of colleges of pharmacy to the number of university health science centers now able and willing to undertake pharmacy education would, in all probability, substantially reduce the number of pharmacists being graduated. It is the opinion of the Study Commission that any significant decrease in the number of well-educated pharmacists would not be in the public interest. A growing population with universal access to and making greater use of health services, an increasing use of drug therapy as a modality of care and treatment, the appearance of new drugs some of which will be used to maintain health, together may greatly increase the demand for pharmacy services and possibly require more pharmacists to provide them.

The problem remains as to how the environment for pharmacy education can be brought to a more satisfactory level in those colleges which are not or cannot immediately become integral parts of a university health science center. Some colleges located in a metropolitan area may be able to associate themselves with health centers and gain access to situations where other health professionals are being educated and health services are being delivered. Some colleges are not so situated or may not be able to effectuate such an association. However, there is good pharmacy practice in many community hospitals. There is good pharmacy practice in many community pharmacies. There is good pharmacy practice in ambulatory clinics of several kinds. In any case, if colleges of pharmacy are to continue they must avail themselves of the facilities required for the basic and generic education of pharmacists at least to the first level of the component objectives of pharmacy education as described in Chapter X.

Training for the generic skills can be given in alternative practice settings. One should be able to learn the basic skills of dispensing equally well in a community pharmacy, in a hospital pharmacy, or in an ambulatory clinic. One should be able to learn the basic skills of communicating with patients and other health professionals in any of these service situations. The same is true for learning the basic skills of keeping and interpreting patient drug records. The same is true in learning the rudiments of organization and management. Thus, it seems that an environment, appropriate to the basic education, can be provided in several alternative ways. However, such environments are not satisfactory for education for any substantial number of differentiations. Certainly in such case no programs beyond the baccalaureate should be attempted and no advanced degrees offered.

This recommendation is not intended to, nor—in the opinion of the Study Commission—does it, limit the opportunities of students of pharmacy to continue their formal education or to obtain training in those differentiated roles requiring additional knowledge and/or skill. It is not necessary that all students receive postgraduate education or training at the institution in which they receive undergraduate education. In fact, there are sound educational reasons why they may not. The number of institutions capable of giving advanced instruction is probably adequate to meet the need. As students choose to progress to higher and more sophisticated pharmacy education they need more complete and more scholarly educational facilities and environments such as are found in university health science centers. Just as the number of graduate schools is far less than the number of undergraduate schools, so should the number of colleges of pharmacy presenting the full range of pharmacy education be less than the number offering the first professional degree.

XIII. CREDENTIALLING IN PHARMACY EDUCATION

No study of a particular professional educational system would be complete without consideration of the credentialling system of that profession. Credentialling takes three forms. First, there is the investigation and monitoring of standards of quality of the educational institutions through the mechanism of accreditation. In pharmacy, accreditation is performed by the American Council for Pharmaceutical Education. This body represents the educational institutions through the American Association of Colleges of Pharmacy, the state boards of pharmacy through the National Association of Boards of Pharmacy, the profession through the American Pharmaceutical Association, and higher education through the American Council on Education. Second, there is certification of the minimum competence of the individual professional through licensure or registration. In pharmacy, licensure or registration is granted by the several state boards of pharmacy. Although each state board is autonomous there is substantial collaboration through their national association. Thus, reciprocity of licensure is facilitated and national standards encouraged. Third, there is certification of competence of those differentiated or specialized individuals who have pursued advanced training and education by voluntary boards representing that differentiated portion of the practicing profession. In pharmacy, differentiation by advanced training has not developed as it has in medicine. Hence, there are presently no specialty boards functioning and no pharmacists are being certified as specialists. However, there is strong interest in certification in several areas of pharmacy. The near future will certainly bring serious proposals to define differentiation, to set up boards, and to begin certification.

The National Association of Boards of Pharmacy is a vigorous organization interested in the advancement of the standards of pharmacy practice through improved licensure practices. The American Council for Pharmaceutical Education is actively studying its accrediting procedures and recently has made an important change. In the past it has accredited colleges of pharmacy. In the future it will accredit programs of pharmacy education.

In all the processes of credentialling—accreditation, licensure, or certification—there is one common mechanism that is necessary for the discharge of these responsibilities. That mechanism is a reliable and widely supported examination system. The state boards of pharmacy rely upon examinations to determine fitness for licensure. If, in the future, there is to be the procedure of relicensure, to give the public assurance of continued competence, it will surely rely upon examinations as well. Accreditation of colleges of pharmacy would be greatly facilitated if the students in all colleges were being evaluated by a national examination. One evidence of the quality of an educational program is the performance of its graduates in comparison to a national standard. The certification of the competence of those profession-als who have acquired additional and differentiated knowledge and skills is wholly dependent upon reliable examinations.

Observation of the several health professions leads to the conclusion that the development of a strong examining system has contributed greatly to the rising quality of education and thereby to an improved and more benefi-cial professional practice. The ultimate result is that the public is better served. It is reasonable to assume that the public would receive improved pharmacy services if there were a national examining system to assist in all the aspects of credentialling.

The National Association of Boards of Pharmacy has taken the first step toward a national examination program. Several years ago a "Blue Ribbon" committee was asked to develop an examination. It is reported that the ex-amination which was produced has been used with some satisfaction by a majority of state boards for licensure determination in their respective juris-dictions. However, the test results have not been made available to the col-leges of pharmacy for self-assessment purposes and are not yet a part of the accrediting process of pharmacy education. There has been active discus-sion of certification of pharmacists practicing in differentiated and more highly skilled roles. In all discussions there is recognition that examinations will have to be developed and administered to serve as a basis of certifica-tion. The development of reliable examinations requires a high degree of specialized and expert knowledge and experience. Psychometry is develop-ing into a science. The development of an examining system is time-con-suming and an expensive process. There are important economies to be made in developing one national system rather than one for each of the states and jurisdictions as well as one for each of the several differentiations which may enter the field of certification.

It is the opinion of the Study Commission that the advisability and the feasibility of developing a national examining system for pharmacy should be promptly and carefully studied. The Commission therefore recommends that the National Association of Boards of Pharmacy, the American Council on Pharmaceutical Education, the American Association of Colleges of Pharmacy, and those professional organizations which are contemplating certification, join in the formation of a committee to study the necessity and the feasibility of creating a National Board of Pharmacy Examiners and to recommend appropriate functions, activities, and organization.

XIV. SUMMARY OF CONCEPTS, FINDINGS,
AND RECOMMENDATIONS

1. The Study Commission recognizes that among deficiencies in the health care system, one is the unavailability of adequate information for those who consume, prescribe, dispense, and administer drugs. This deficiency has resulted in inappropriate drug use and an unacceptable frequency of drug-induced disease. Pharmacists are seen as health professionals who could make an important contribution to the health care system of the future by providing information about drugs to consumers and health professionals. Education and training of pharmacists now and in the future must be developed to meet these important responsibilities.

2. The Study Commission advances the concept that pharmacy should be conceived basically as a *knowledge system* which renders a *health service* by concerning itself with understanding drugs and their effects upon people and animals. Pharmacy generates knowledge about drugs, acquires relevant knowledge from the biological, chemical, physical, and behavioral sciences; it tests, organizes, and applies that knowledge. Pharmacy translates a substantial portion of that knowledge into drug products and distributes them widely to those who require them. Pharmacy knowledge is disseminated to physicians, pharmacists, and other health professionals and to the general public to the end that drug knowledge and products may contribute to the health of individuals and the welfare of society (cf. pp. 11-14) [pp. 153-156].*

3. The Study Commission believes that a pharmacist must be defined as an individual who is engaged in *one of the steps of a system called pharmacy.* We cannot define a pharmacist simply as one who practices pharmacy. Rather, he must be defined as one who practices a part of pharmacy which is determined by the activities carried on in one of the subsystems of pharmacy. A pharmacist is characterized by the common denominator of drug knowledge and *the differentiated additional* knowledge and skill required by his particular role (cf. pp. 28-30) [pp. 163-165].

4. The Study Commission believes that the system of pharmacy must be described as being both effective and efficient in developing, manufacturing, and distributing drug products. However, the system of pharmacy cannot be described at present as either effective or efficient in developing, organizing, and distributing *knowledge and information* about drugs. When pharmacy is viewed as a knowledge system, it must be judged as only partially successful in delivering its full potential as a health service to the members of society (cf. pp. 56-59) [pp. 183-184].

5. The Study Commission recommends that major attention be given to the problems of drug information to find who needs to know, what he needs

---

*Bracketed pagination refers to pages in Appendix A.

to know, and how these needs can best be met with speed and economy (cf. p. 55) [p. 182].

6. It is the opinion of the Study Commission that in spite of the real and multifaceted differentiation in the practice roles of pharmacists, there is a common body of knowledge, skill, attitudes, and behavior which all pharmacists must possess. In a practical and detailed sense the objectives of pharmacy education must be stated in terms of *both the common knowledge and skill and of the differentiated and/or additional knowledge and skill required for specific practice roles.* This can be done only by starting a series of limited educational objectives, which if met in sequential order will accomplish both common and differentiated objectives (cf. p. 109) [pp. 215-216].

7. The Study Commission recommends the following three component educational objectives for pharmacy education:

    a. The mastery of the knowledge and the acquisition of the skills which are *common* to all of the roles of pharmacy practice.

    b. The mastery of the additional knowledge and the acquisition of the additional skill needed for those differentiated roles which require additional *pharmacy* knowledge and experience.

    c. The mastery of the additional knowledge and the acquisition of the additional skills needed for those differentiated roles which require additional knowledge and skill *other than pharmacy* (cf. pp. 109-112) [pp. 215-218].

8. The Study Commission recommends that every school of pharmacy promptly find the ways and means to provide appropriate practice opportunities for its faculty members having clinical teaching responsibilities so that they may serve as effective role models for their students (cf. pp. 114-115) [p. 219].

9. It is the opinion of the Study Commission that the curricula of the schools of pharmacy should be based upon the *competencies* desired for their graduates rather than upon the basis of knowledge available in the several relevant sciences (cf. p. 123) [p. 224].

10. It is the opinion of the Study Commission that the greatest weakness of the schools of pharmacy is a lack of an adequate number of *clinical scientists* who can relate their specialized scientific knowledge to the development of the practice skills required to provide effective, efficient, and needed patient services. The Study Commission recommends that support be sought for a program to train a modest number of clinical scientists for pharmacy education (cf. pp. 123-126) [pp. 224-225].

11. The Study Commission emphasizes that pharmacy is a knowledge system in which *chemical substances and people called patients* interact. Needed and optimally effective drug therapy results only when drugs and those who consume them are fully understood. We suggest that one of the

first steps in reviewing the educational program of a college of pharmacy should be weighing the relative emphasis given to the physical and biological sciences against the behavioral and social sciences in the curriculum for the first professional degree. (cf. pp. 101 and 126-127) [pp. 210-211 and 225-226].

12. The Study Commission believes that those schools of pharmacy with adequate resources should develop, in addition to the first professional degree, programs of instruction at the graduate and advanced professional level for more differentiated roles of pharmacy practice (cf. pp. 129-132) [pp. 229-231].

13. It is the opinion of the Study Commission that the optimal environment for pharmacy education is the university health science center for the full range of knowledge, skill, and practice can be found there. However, the Commission does not believe that it is practical or in the public interest to recommend that all colleges of pharmacy must be so located. Alternative arrangements, if effectively utilized, can provide an acceptable environment for the education of students at the baccalaureate level (cf. pp. 129-132) [pp. 229-231].

14. It is the opinion of the Study Commission that all aspects of credentialling of pharmacists and pharmacy education and the quality of pharmacy education would be enhanced by the services of a National Board of Pharmacy Examiners. The Commission recommends that the National Association of Boards of Pharmacy, the American Council on Pharmaceutical Education, the American Association of Colleges of Pharmacy and those professional organizations contemplating specialty certification, join in the formation of a committee to study the necessity and the feasibility of creating a National Board of Pharmacy Examiners and to recommend appropriate functions, activities, and organization (cf. pp. 135-138) [pp. 233-234].

FOOTNOTES

Chapter I

1. Cluff, L. E., Caranosos, G. J., Stewart, R. B.: *Clinical Problems With Drugs,* W. B. Saunders Company, Philadelphia, 1975, pp. 10, 11.

Chapter III

2. Rodowskas, C. A., Jr., Director, Dickson, W. M., Assistant Director, Pharmacy Manpower Information Project, American Association of Colleges of Pharmacy, 1971-1975. (Supported by the Bureau of Health Manpower, Health Resources Administration, Department of Health Education and Welfare.)

Chapter V

3. *Research and Development in Industry,* 1971, National Science Foundation, Surveys of Science Resources Series, No. 73-305, Washington, DC, 1973.

Chapter VII

4. *Population Estimates and Projections,* Current Population Reports, Series R. 25, No. 541, Department of Commerce, Bureau of the Census, Washington, DC, 1975.

5. *Final Report,* Task Force on Prescription Drugs, Department of Health, Education, and Welfare, Washington, DC, 1969, p. 1.

Chapter VIII

6. Elliott, Edward C., Director, *The General Report of the Pharmaceutical Survey, 1946-1949,* American Council on Education, Washington, DC, 1950.

CONSULTANTS TO THE STUDY COMMISSION ON PHARMACY

Consultant	Category of Consultation
John G. Adams, PhD Vice President, Office of Scientific and Professional Relations Pharmaceutical Manufacturers Association Washington, DC	Pharmaceutical Associations
William S. Apple, PhD Executive Director American Pharmaceutical Association Washington, DC	Pharmaceutical Associations
Myrtle K. Aydelotte, PhD Director, Department of Nursing University of Iowa Hospitals and Clinics Iowa City, Iowa	Hospital Nursing Practice
C. E. Barnett, JD Chairman, Executive Committee National Association of Boards of Pharmacy Now: Executive Secretary Idaho Board of Pharmacy Boise, Idaho	Pharmacy Licensure
William H. Barr, PhD Professor and Chairman Department of Pharmacy and Pharmaceutics Health Sciences Division Virginia Commonwealth University Richmond, Virginia	Pharmaceutical Education
Thomas G. Bidder, MD Associate Professor Pharmacology and Psychiatry School of Medicine Case Western Reserve University Cleveland, Ohio Now:	Medical Education and Practice

Department of Psychiatry
VA Hospital
Supulveda, California

Leland B. Blanchard, MD   Medical Education
Clinical Associate Professor   and Practice
Department of Medicine
Department of Family, Community,
    and Preventive Medicine
Stanford University
Stanford, California

Ralph N. Blomster, PhD   Pharmaceutical
Professor and Chairman   Education
Department of Pharmacognosy
School of Pharmacy
University of Maryland
Baltimore, Maryland

Ralph C. Boehm, MS, Pharmacy   Federal Hospital
Deputy Director of Pharmacy Services   Pharmacy Practice
Veterans Administration
Washington, DC
    Now:
Chief, Pharmacy Services
VA Hospital
San Diego, California

Michael Bongiovanni, BS   Pharmaceutical
President, U.S. Pharmaceutical Company   Industry
E. R. Squibb & Sons, Inc.
Princeton, New Jersey

Lawrence R. Borgsdorff, PharmD   Clinical Pharmacy
Docent Clinical Pharmacist   Practice
Kansas City General Hospital
    and Medical Center,
and Associate Professor of Clinical Pharmacy
School of Pharmacy and Medicine
University of Missouri
Kansas City, Missouri

Allen J. Brands, DSc   Federal Participation
Pharmacy Liaison Officer   in Pharmacy
Public Health Service
Department of Health, Education, and Welfare
Rockville, Maryland

W. Paul Briggs, EdD   Pharmaceutical
Executive Director Emeritus   Associations
American Foundation
   for Pharmaceutical Education
Washington, DC

Donald C. Brodie, PhD   Pharmaceutical
Adjunct Professor of Medicine and Pharmacy   Education
Schools of Medicine and Pharmacy
University of Southern California
Los Angeles, California

C. J. Cavallito, PhD   Pharmaceutical
Executive Vice President   Industry
Scientific Affairs
Ayerst Laboratories
New York, New York

Frazier Cheston   Pharmaceutical
Vice President   Industry
Director of Customer Affairs
Menley & James Laboratories
Division, SmithKline Corporation
Philadelphia, Pennsylvania

Bernard E. Conley, PhD   Federal Participation
Chief, Drug Utilization Studies Program   in Pharmacy
Health Resources Administration
Department of Health, Education, and Welfare
Rockville, Maryland

Albert A. Cook, BS, Pharmacy   Hospital Pharmacy
Director of Pharmacy   Practice
Reid Memorial Hospital
Richmond, Indiana

Salvatore J. D'Angelo, BS, Pharmacy
Member, Executive Committee
National Association of Retail Druggists
New Orleans, Louisiana

Pharmaceutical
Associations

Robert A. Danielson, MD
Assistant Professor, Surgery
School of Medicine
Case Western Reserve University
Cleveland, Ohio

Medical Education
and Practice

George W. Drach, MD
Associate Professor of Surgery/Urology
and Chief of Urology
College of Medicine
University of Arizona
Tucson, Arizona

Medical Education
and Practice

Frederick M. Eckel, MS
Associate Professor, Hospital Pharmacy
School of Pharmacy
University of North Carolina
Chapel Hill, North Carolina

Nursing Home
Practice

Paul M. Eicher, MD
Chairman, Department of Pediatrics
Lovelace-Bataan Medical Center
and Associate Clinical Professor, Pediatrics
University of New Mexico
Albuquerque, New Mexico

Medical Education
and Practice

John J. Fenstermacher, BS
Senior Vice President—Retail Sales
McKesson & Robbins Drug Company
San Francisco, California

Pharmaceutical
Industry

Kenneth F. Finger, PhD
Associate Vice President
    for Health Affairs
and Dean, College of Pharmacy
University of Florida
Gainesville, Florida

Pharmaceutical
Education

Albert B. Fisher Jr., PhD   Pharmaceutical
President   Associations
American Foundation for Pharmaceutical
    Education
Fair Lawn, New Jersey

William L. Ford, BA   Pharmaceutical
Executive Vice President   Associations
National Wholesale Druggists Association
Scarsdale, New York

Thomas O. Fox, BS, Pharmacy   Community Pharmacy
Owner, Prescription Arts Pharmacies   Practice
Detroit, Michigan

Vincent Gardner, MBA   Federal Participation
Chief, Drug Studies Branch   in Pharmacy
Social Security Administration
Department of Health, Education, and Welfare
Washington, DC

Alan L. Gordon, MD   Medical Education
Medical Specialists, Ltd.   and Practice
Phoenix, Arizona

Raymond A. Gosselin, ScD   Pharmaceutical
President   Education
Massachusetts College of Pharmacy
Boston, Massachusetts

Gordon F. Goyette Jr., BS, Pharmacy   Pharmaceutical
Director, Public Affairs   Industry
Parke, Davis & Company
Detroit, Michigan

Melvin W. Green, PhD   Accreditation
Director Emeritus of Educational Relations   of Schools
American Council on Pharmaceutical Education   of Pharmacy
Southport, North Carolina

Paul Grussing, BS, Pharmacy   Pharmacy Licensure
Externship Coordinator
College of Pharmacy
University of Minnesota

and Executive Secretary
Minnesota Board of Pharmacy
Minneapolis, Minnesota

Philip D. Hansten, PharmD   Pharmaceutical
Assistant Professor, Clinical Pharmacy   Education
College of Pharmacy
Washington State University
Pullman, Washington

Donald C. Harrington, MD   Medical Foundation
Medical Director   Practice
Foundation for Medical Care
   of San Joaquin County
Stockton, California

Berel Held, MD   Medical Education
Professor and Chairman   and Practice
Department of Obstetrics and Gynecology
University of Texas Medical School—Houston
Houston, Texas

Rex C. Higley, BS   Pharmacy Licensure
Director, Bureau of Examining Boards
Department of Health, Nebraska
Lincoln, Nebraska

Charles A. Hughes, BS, Pharmacy   Pharmacy Licensure
Owner and Operator, Hughes Pharmacy
and Chairman, Iowa Board of Pharmacy
Emmetsburg, Iowa

Daniel A. Hussar, PhD   Pharmaceutical
Professor and Director   Education
Department of Pharmacy
  Now:
Dean, Philadelphia College of Pharmacy
  and Science
Philadelphia, Pennsylvania

Richard A. Jackson, PhD   Pharmaceutical
Assistant Professor of Health Care   Education
  Administration

Southern School of Pharmacy
Mercer University
Atlanta, Georgia

M. T. Jenkins, MD   Medical Education
McDermott Professor and Chairman   and Practice
Department of Anesthesiology
University of Texas Southwestern Medical
    School and
Parkland Memorial Hospital
Dallas, Texas

David A. Knapp, PhD   Pharmaceutical
Professor, Pharmacy Administration   Education
School of Pharmacy
University of Maryland
Baltimore, Maryland

Frank E. Kunkel, PhC   Pharmacy Licensure
Executive Director
Ohio State Board of Pharmacy
Columbus, Ohio

Bernard J. Lachner, MBA   Hospital
President and Chief Executive Officer   Administration
Evanston Hospital
and Professor of Management
Graduate School of Management
Northwestern University
Evanston, Illinois

Jules B. LaPidus, PhD   Pharmaceutical
Vice Provost and Dean   Education
The Graduate School
Ohio State University
Columbus, Ohio

Irwin Lerner, MBA   Pharmaceutical
Group Vice President   Industry
Hoffman-LaRoche, Inc.
Nutley, New Jersey

Fred T. Mahaffey, PharmD   Pharmacy Licensure
Executive Director
National Association of Boards of Pharmacy
and Secretary, American Council
    on Pharmaceutical Education
Chicago, Illinois

Robert F. Maronde, MD   Ambulatory Care
Professor of Medicine   Practice
Head, Clinical Pharmacology Section
School of Medicine
University of Southern California
Los Angeles, California

Kathleen McGee, BS, Pharmacy   Pharmaceutical
Director of Professional Services   Associations
National Association of Chain Drug Stores
Arlington, Virginia

Peter D. Meister, PhD   Pharmaceutical
Director, Supportive Research   Industry
The Upjohn Company
Kalamazoo, Michigan

Kenneth L. Melmon, MD   Medical Education
Professor of Medicine and Pharmacology   and Practice
Chief, Division of Clinical Pharmacology
University of California Medical Center
San Franciso, California

J. Chris Mitsuoka, PharmD   Pharmacy Student
Resident in Clinical Pharmacy
School of Pharmacy
University of California
San Francisco, California

Daniel J. Nona, PhD   Pharmacy Licensure
Professor of Pharmacy
College of Pharmacy
University of Illinois
    Now:
Director of Educational Relations

American Council on Pharmaceutical
   Education
Chicago, Illinois

Mark Novitch, MD   Federal Participation
Deputy Associate Commissioner   in Pharmacy
   for Medical Affairs
Food and Drug Administration
Department of Health, Education, and Welfare
Rockville, Maryland

Phillip M. Nudelman, BS, Pharmacy   Group Health Care
Director of Paramedical Services   Practice
   and Pharmacy Services
Group Health Cooperative of Puget Sound
Seattle, Washington

Joseph A. Oddis, DSc   Pharmaceutical
Executive Director   Associations
American Society of Hospital Pharmacists
Bethesda, Maryland

Paul F. Parker, MS   Pharmaceutical
Professor of Pharmacy   Education
College of Pharmacy
University of Kentucky
Lexington, Kentucky

Robert E. Pearson, MS, Pharmacy   Drug Information
Acting Chairman and Associate Professor Practice
Department of Pharmacy
State University of New York at Buffalo
Buffalo, New York

Cornelius W. Pettinga, PhD   Pharmaceutical
Executive Vice President   Industry
Eli Lilly & Company
Indianapolis, Indiana

John Ruggiero, PhD   Pharmaceutical
Assistant Vice President   Associations
Office of Scientific and Professional Relations
and Director of Pharmacy Relations

Pharmaceutical Manufacturers Association
Washington, DC

George L. Scharringhausen Jr., PhC   Community Pharmacy
President   Practice
Scharringhausen Pharmacy, Inc.
Park Ridge, Illinois

Alexander Schmidt, MD   Federal Participation
Commissioner   in Pharmacy
Food and Drug Administration
Department of Health, Education, and Welfare
Rockville, Maryland

Doris Schwartz, MA   Public Health Nursing
Associate Professor of Nursing   Practice
Cornell University/New York Hospital
    School of Nursing
New York, New York

Joe Schwemin, BS   Pharmacy Licensure
President
National Association of Boards of Pharmacy
    Now:
Executive Secretary-Director
Oklahoma State Board of Pharmacy
Oklahoma City, Oklahoma

Henry Simmons, MD   Federal Participation
Former Deputy Assistant Secretary for Health in Pharmacy
Department of Health, Education, and Welfare
Washington, DC

Henry Spiegelblatt, MPA   Federal Participation
Director, Division of Policy and Standards   in Pharmacy
Medical Service Administration
Department of Health, Education, and Welfare
Washington, DC

C. Joseph Stetler, LLB   Pharmaceutical
President   Associations
Pharmaceutical Manufacturers Association
Washington, DC

John H. Stocking, MS, Hospital Administration   Mental Hospital
Administrator   Administration
Anoka State Hospital
Anoka, Minnesota

Cindy Tasset, BS, Pharmacy   Pharmacy Student
Chairperson, AACP Council of Students
and Student at School of Pharmacy
University of Kansas
Lawrence, Kansas
    Now:
Pharmacist, Baker Messer Drug Store
Pratt, Kansas

Varro E. Tyler, PhD   Accreditation
Dean   of Schools
School of Pharmacy and Pharmacal Sciences   of Pharmacy
Purdue University
Lafayette, Indiana,
and President
American Council on Pharmaceutical
    Education

James N. Tyson, MS   Pharmaceutical
Executive Secretary   Associations
National Pharmaceutical Association,
    Inc., and
Associate Professor of Pharmacy
College of Pharmacy
Howard University
Washington, DC

Charles A. Walton, PhD   Pharmaceutical
Assistant Dean   Education
and Professor of Pharmacology
    and Clinical Pharmacy
College of Pharmacy
University of Texas at Austin
Austin, Texas

Nathan Watzman, PhD   Federal Participation
Chief, Optometry, Pharmacy, Podiatry   in Pharmacy
    and Veterinary Medicine

Education Branch
Health Resources Administration
  Now:
Acting Associate Director
Division of Associated Health Programs
Bureau of Health Manpower
Department of Health, Education, and Welfare
Bethesda, Maryland

Paul F. Wehrle, MD   Medical Education
Hastings Professor of Pediatrics   and Practice
University of Southern California
and Chief, Professional Services, Department
    of Pediatrics
Los Angeles County/University of
    Southern California Medical Center
Los Angeles, California

M. Keith Weikel, PhD   Federal Participation
Acting Associate Administrator   in Pharmacy
    for Planning Evaluation and Legislation
Health Resources Administration
  Now:
Commissioner of Medical Service
    Administration, Social and Rehabilitation
    Services
Department of Health, Education, and Welfare
Washington, DC

Jean K. Weston, MD   Pharmacology
President   Research
Weston Research Laboratories, Inc.
Purcellville, Virginia

Maxwell M. Wintrobe, MD, PhD   Medical Education
Distinguished Professor of Internal Medicine   and Practice
College of Medicine
University of Utah
Salt Lake City, Utah

Gerald C. Wojta   Pharmaceutical
President   Industry
Philips Roxane Laboratories, Inc.

(subsidiary of North American Philips
    Corporation)
Columbus, Ohio

William E. Woods, JD   Pharmaceutical
Washington Representative   Associations
and Associate General Counsel
National Association of Retail Druggists
Washington, DC

Michael Zagorac, MBA   Pharmaceutical
Vice President   Associations
National Association of Chain Drug Stores
Arlington, Virginia

Appendix B

Twentieth-Century Pharmacy Studies

From the beginning of the twentieth century until the publication of *Pharmacists for the Future,* there were a number of studies that focused on pharmacy and pharmacists. Some of these, such as the *General Report of the Pharmaceutical Survey,* looked broadly at the profession. Others, such as the *Pharmaceutical Curriculum* or the *Mirror to Hospital Pharmacy,* looked at a single aspect or a practice site.

Almost every study required significant efforts by the profession, first to fund and then to complete. At least one of the objectives in almost every study was to determine what had to be done to help the profession, either immediately or in the future, and determine how to do it. Many included education either as the object of the study or as part of the recommendation.

Most studies focused on the profession. That is, they examined the profession and its different components. Only a few later studies addressed what the profession was supposed to deliver to the patient, the customer of the profession. This shift began to occur with the interest in clinical pharmacy and culminated in the Millis Commission.

These studies are signposts to the maturation of a profession and professional education during the greater part of a century.

SURVEYS AND CONFERENCES 1905-1975

Date	Title	Author	Sponsor
1905	Scoville Report	Scoville, Wilbur L.	American Conference of Pharmaceutical Faculties
1924	The Charters Study	Charters, W.W.	American Conference of Pharmaceutical Faculties

1932	Cost of Medicines: The Manufacture and Distribution of Drugs and Medicines in the United States and the Services of Pharmacy in Medical Care	Rorem, C. Rufus and Fischelis, Robert P.	Committee on the Costs of Medical Care
1933	The Prescription Ingredient Survey	Gathercoal, E.N.	American Pharmaceutical Association
1942	Bernays Survey	Bernays, Edward L.	
1945	The Independent Druggist, Report #1		National Association of Retail Druggists and The Saturday Evening Post
1947	The Independent Druggist, Report #2		National Association of Retail Druggists and The Saturday Evening Post
1950	The General Report of the Pharmaceutical Survey: 1946-49	Elliott, Edward C.	American Council on Education
1952	The Pharmaceutical Curriculum	Blauch, Lloyd E. and Webster, George L.	Committee on Curriculum, American Association of Colleges of Pharmacy
1960	Liberal Education and Pharmacy	Newcomer, James, Bunnell, Kevin P., and McGrath, Earl J.	Institute of Higher Education
1961	Survey of Retail Pharmacists	Benson & Benson, Inc.	Readers Digest
1963	Mirror to Hospital Pharmacy	Francke, Don E., Latiolais, Clifton J., Francke, Gloria N., and Ho, Norman F.H.	American Society of Hospital Pharmacists
1965	Exploratory Paper for a Proposed National Study of Pharmacy as a Professional Occupation	Sonnedecker, Glenn A.	American Pharmaceutical Association
1966	The Challenge to Pharmacy in Times of Change: A Report of the Commission on Pharmaceutical Services to Ambulatory Patients by Hospitals and Related Facilities	Brodie, Donald C.	American Pharmaceutical Association and The American Society of Hospital Pharmacists

Year	Study	Author	Organization
1967	Pharmacy-Medicine-Nursing Conference on Health Education	Deno, Richard A.	University of Michigan College of Pharmacy, Medical School and School of Nursing
1968	Task Force on Prescription Drugs	Subcommittee on Monopoly of the Select Committee on Small Business, United States Senate	U.S. Department of Health, Education, and Welfare
1969	Proceedings of the Third Professional Pharmacy Seminar	DeBoest, Henry F.	Eli Lilly Company
1970	Challenge to Pharmacy in the 70s: Proceedings of an Invitational Conference on Pharmacy Manpower	Graber, Joe B. and Brodie, Donald C.	School of Pharmacy, University of California–San Francisco and National Center for Health Services Research and Development
1971	ASHP-AACP Invitational Workshop on Clinical Pharmaceutical Practice and Education		American Society of Hospital Pharmacists and American Association of Colleges of Pharmacy
1972	Educating for the Health Team: Report of a Conference	Conference on the Interrelationships of Educational Programs for Health Professionals	National Academy of Sciences, Institute of Medicine
1972	Pharmacy Manpower Information Project	Rodowskas, Christopher J. and Dickson, W. Michael	American Association of Colleges of Pharmacy
1972	Clinical Pharmacy Education and Training Program: A Special Report	Skinner, William J.	American Association of Colleges of Pharmacy
1973	Evaluating Pharmacists and Their Activities	Knapp, David A. and Smith, Mickey C.	American Society of Hospital Pharmacists
1973	Study of Costs of Educating Health Professionals by the Institute of Medicine, National Academy of Science		

| 1973 | Communicating the Value of Comprehensive Pharmaceutical Services to the Consumer | The Dichter Institute for Motivational Research, Inc. | American Pharmaceutical Association |
| 1975 | Pharmacists for the Future: The Report of the Study Commission on Pharmacy | Millis, John S. | American Association of Colleges of Pharmacy |

Index

Page numbers followed by the letter "t" indicate tables.

Order a copy of this book with this form or online at:
http://www.haworthpress.com/store/product.asp?sku=5151

THE MILLIS STUDY COMMISSION ON PHARMACY
A Road Map to a Profession's Future

_____ in hardbound at $59.95 (ISBN-13: 978-0-7890-2424-4; ISBN-10: 0-7890-2424-1)

_____ in softbound at $39.95 (ISBN-13: 978-0-7890-2425-1; ISBN-10: 0-7890-2425-X)

Or order online and use special offer code HEC25 in the shopping cart.

COST OF BOOKS_____

POSTAGE & HANDLING_____
(US: $4.00 for first book & $1.50
for each additional book)
(Outside US: $5.00 for first book
& $2.00 for each additional book)

SUBTOTAL_____

IN CANADA: ADD 7% GST_____

STATE TAX_____
(NJ, NY, OH, MN, CA, IL, IN, PA, & SD
residents, add appropriate local sales tax)

FINAL TOTAL_____
(If paying in Canadian funds,
convert using the current
exchange rate, UNESCO
coupons welcome)

☐ **BILL ME LATER:** (Bill-me option is good on
US/Canada/Mexico orders only; not good to
jobbers, wholesalers, or subscription agencies.)
☐ Check here if billing address is different from
shipping address and attach purchase order and
billing address information.

Signature_____

☐ **PAYMENT ENCLOSED: $**_____

☐ **PLEASE CHARGE TO MY CREDIT CARD.**

☐ Visa ☐ MasterCard ☐ AmEx ☐ Discover
☐ Diner's Club ☐ Eurocard ☐ JCB

Account # _____

Exp. Date_____

Signature_____

Prices in US dollars and subject to change without notice.

NAME_____

INSTITUTION_____

ADDRESS_____

CITY_____

STATE/ZIP_____

COUNTRY_____ COUNTY (NY residents only)_____

TEL_____ FAX_____

E-MAIL_____

May we use your e-mail address for confirmations and other types of information? ☐ Yes ☐ No
We appreciate receiving your e-mail address and fax number. Haworth would like to e-mail or fax special
discount offers to you, as a preferred customer. **We will never share, rent, or exchange your e-mail address
or fax number.** We regard such actions as an invasion of your privacy.

Order From Your Local Bookstore or Directly From
The Haworth Press, Inc.
10 Alice Street, Binghamton, New York 13904-1580 • USA
TELEPHONE: 1-800-HAWORTH (1-800-429-6784) / Outside US/Canada: (607) 722-5857
FAX: 1-800-895-0582 / Outside US/Canada: (607) 771-0012
E-mail to: orders@haworthpress.com

For orders outside US and Canada, you may wish to order through your local
sales representative, distributor, or bookseller.
For information, see http://haworthpress.com/distributors

(Discounts are available for individual orders in US and Canada only, not booksellers/distributors.)
PLEASE PHOTOCOPY THIS FORM FOR YOUR PERSONAL USE.
http://www.HaworthPress.com   BOF04